The Baby Cookbook
Revised Edition

THE BABY COOKBOOK

Revised Edition

*Tasty and Nutritious Meals
for the Whole Family That
Babies and Toddlers Will Also Love*

KARIN KNIGHT, R.N.,
AND JEANNIE LUMLEY

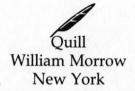

Quill
William Morrow
New York

It is the policy of William Morrow and Company, Inc., and its imprints and affiliates, recognizing the importance of preserving what has been written, to print the books we publish on acid-free paper, and we exert our best efforts to that end.

Library of Congress Cataloging-in-Publication Data

Knight, Karin.
    The baby cookbook / Karin Knight and Jeannie Lumley.—Rev. ed.
      p.   cm.
    ISBN 0-688-10358-8
    1. Cookery (Baby foods) 2. Infants—Nutrition. I. Lumley,
Jeannie. II. Title.
TX740.K59   1991b
649'.3—dc20   92-867
                                                     CIP

Printed in the United States of America

6 7 8 9 10

BOOK DESIGN BY ARLENE SCHLEIFER GOLDBERG

To my beloved Baba, Muktananda
—K.K.

Foreword

FROM a practical standpoint, the feeding of infants and young children presents a number of challenges to young parents. Our society has changed from the days of the close family unit, when experienced grandparents were available to give counsel. Young couples are left primarily to "on-the-job training" in deciding what is best in child rearing. Good pediatric care and evaluation, with advice on such basic information as healthy nutrition, can be costly or unavailable, for many parents. Unfortunately, even where such care is available, many times a good, healthy nutritional program is not a major part of the care provided.

We have come to new understandings of the importance of healthy nutrition in recent years. More and more young parents are seeking to learn how best to feed their children and to be models of good eating habits themselves.

The Baby Cookbook is a valuable, readable guide to basic nutritional facts, set in the context of feeding an infant from the introduction of early solids at approximately six months of age to the time of independent self-feeding and diet selection by the age of two years. Both the principles of sound nutrition and a reasonable, practical approach to when, how, and what to offer a child at each stage of his development are covered. The progression from puréed to more coarse (junior texture) foods through to soft table foods and finger-feeding of small pieces of table foods is appropriately detailed. The many recipes, which can be prepared, stored, and served by the busy parent inexpensively and conveniently, make this book a complete, practical guide to feeding children during their first two years.

With this book Karin Knight and Jeannie Lumley have made a significant contribution to parents and their young children, and they have provided as well a referral source for physicians in this important area of good nutrition. Equally valuable is their approach to the hows and whys of developing good patterns and habits of feeding, which are often so difficult for new parents to establish.

H. JAMES HOLROYD, M.D., F.A.A.P.
Clinical Professor of Pediatrics
University of Southern California
School of Medicine

Foreword

The Baby Cookbook is an excellent resource for new parents who are faced with the task of providing a healthy diet for their children. Karin Knight has sorted through the myriad of nutrition myths and misconceptions to compile a concise, accurate, and informative handbook on the hows and whys of nourishing both infant and toddler.

The thoughts recorded in the diary section will help parents reflect on the challenges they face at each stage of the child's development.

A wide selection of low-salt, low-sugar recipes offers many inspirations to end the "What shall I cook today?" doldrums. There are numerous recipes that the whole family will enjoy, and they wisely incorporate foods from many cultures. Exposing the young child to a variety of foods will help to mold healthy eating patterns that should last a lifetime.

LINDA BROWN, R.D., M.P.H.
Chief Clinical Dietitian
Children's Hospital of Los Angeles

Contents

PART 1
Nutrition and Feeding Guide
from Six Months to Two Years

PART 2
Family Recipes
and Special Children's Recipes

Introduction

You are probably reading *The Baby Cookbook, Revised Edition* because you are a new parent, or are expecting a baby. And you are obviously anxious to do the best possible job in raising a happy, healthy child. When I was forty-three years old my daughter, Mirabai, was born. Having raised two teenage sons, this seemed a wonderful opportunity to remedy some of the mistakes I had made with them, especially regarding their eating habits. My work as a public health nurse made me very aware of the importance of a nutritious diet for both good childhood development and health in maturity. With this in mind, I kept a diary of Mirabai's progress, from breastfeeding to solids and on to family meals. This diary eventually became the foundation for *The Baby Cookbook*.

Observing my daughter, I was amazed to see how quickly both good and bad eating habits were formed. It seemed to me that if healthy eating patterns were established when solids were introduced, most food-related problems that occur later in life could be prevented. Mirabai, who is now a preteen in middle school, is proving this premise. She is remarkably healthy, rarely absent from school, and most of her visits to the doctor are for routine checkups. She is a slim, happy child who chooses balanced and nutritious foods from the school cafeteria and in restaurants as well as at home.

Although there are very few changes to the information included in the first edition of *The Baby Cookbook*, the vitamin and mineral charts have been completely updated. We have also expanded the section on fluoride, a subject that has become a concern to many parents. Following extensive research, the most current information on fluoride is included here in a straightforward way.

As there is also justifiable concern with the problem of childhood obesity, I have added information about cholesterol and eggs, and expanded the segment on fats.

You will find a new chapter on microwave cooking, with lots of information and recipes for infants, toddlers, and family meals, as well as another quick and easy chapter on crockpot cooking, with wonderful meals that cook themselves. All of these are especially valuable to busy parents who are looking to provide delicious and nutritious foods in a minimum amount of time.

There are a few points I must emphasize:

- This is a well-baby book. If you are in any doubt whatsoever about your baby's health, consult a physician.
- Although I recommend starting solids at six months of age, all babies have individual needs. Some may be ready for solids earlier, while others may still be mainly breast-fed at a year. You and your pediatrician should judge when the time is right to change your baby's diet.
- Your observations and instincts about your child are usually best. The information included in this book should be used with that in mind.

A pediatrician recently reminded me that the food we eat and the water we drink are not the pure sources of nourishment they once were. Poisons exist in many of our foods, which should be of real concern to us as parents. If you wish to explore the subject in depth, I recommend reading *Diet for a Poisoned Planet* by David Steinman. It is a sensible guide for safer nutrition for all of us.

As you can see, *The Baby Cookbook, Revised Edition* covers a

wide range of information on raising healthy children. My aim
has been to provide a complete feeding guide in the context
of family life. I hope you will find it of value not only to your
baby or child, but to the general well-being of your entire
family.

—KARIN KNIGHT, R.N.

Part 1

NUTRITION AND FEEDING GUIDE FROM SIX MONTHS TO TWO YEARS

Nutrition and Nutrients—Their Importance to Babies

SAGES have said that food nourishes and protects, and food destroys. Food is life, and food is disease. What we consume should refine our intellect, give us inner peace, keep our mind and body strong, and enable us to function beautifully in life. What better could we want for our babies?

The sages and science seem to think alike here. Most of our illnesses are diet related, especially congestive heart failure, cancer, diabetes, strokes, and heart attacks. Good nutrition will give us good health if we also have a happy, healthy attitude toward our diet and our body. Love, happiness, laughter, and caring—all need to be added to a nutritious diet for total well-being.

Most of us think of diet and nutrition as the same thing. However, diet is the food and liquids we consume (some of which the body uses and some of which go to waste), and nutrition is the process by which the body utilizes what we eat and drink. Food supplies the raw materials for growth and energy. It allows the body to pursue its complicated process of metabolism. All living cells require a multitude of nutrients and may become malnourished if even one essential ingredient is lacking.

Good nutrition is required for normal development in all

children. It also helps maintain the body's natural defense system, which in turn helps the body resist infections. To achieve good nutrition, our bodies need an adequate and balanced amount of protein, fats, carbohydrates, vitamins, and minerals.

A well baby is born with a vibrant, healthy body. As new parents, it is one of our primary duties to maintain our children's good health. The foundations for your baby's future well-being are being laid now, and during these early years you will have the pleasure of watching him develop through one of the most exciting and crucial growth periods of his life. I hope the following pages will help make the experience a joyful and healthy one for both of you.

PROTEINS

Proteins are invaluable. They are necessary for tissue maintenance and repair. They help build blood and antibodies to fight infection and are an important source of energy. They aid healthy digestion and are essential for proper elimination of waste material. A lack of protein may cause a craving for sweets and starches, and protein malnutrition can cause permanent stunting of physical growth, failure to reach full intellectual development, and susceptibility to infectious diseases.

Since the chief function of proteins is to supply the body with building materials, they can be thought of as "building blocks"—in nutritional language, amino acids. The human body is capable of manufacturing fourteen of these amino acids, which are referred to as "nonessential" because they need not be obtained from specific dietary sources. Certain amino acids cannot be manufactured by the body itself, or cannot be formed at a sufficiently rapid rate to meet the body's demands, and are called "essential" amino acids. There are eight of them—lysine, leucine, isoleucine, methionine, tryptophan, threonine, valine, and phenylalanine—all of which must be obtained from food sources.

There are two additional amino acids, histidine and arginine, which may also be called essential for children, as their bodies cannot produce them fast enough to ensure an adequate supply. Both are plentiful in cheese, milk, and eggs.

A "complete protein" must contain all these essential amino acids, the best food sources for which are fish, poultry, meat, eggs, cheese, and milk.

Other foods contain some amino acids but not all, and these foods are called "incomplete proteins." Peas, most kinds of beans, rice, cereals, lentils, and processed flour all provide incomplete proteins. However, if different kinds of incomplete proteins are combined, excellent sources of high complete protein can be created (see table page 25). However, a few points should be kept in mind:

- The importance of knowing which foods complement others. (Sometimes information is limited on amino acid content.)
- A larger quantity of food is necessary to supply adequate amounts of protein from incomplete-protein sources, and children's stomachs and appetites are small.
- A well-balanced meal combining beans and rice, tofu and rice, or beans and pasta will not be adequate if a child will eat only one of the two foods.
- Two or more incomplete proteins *must* be eaten at the same time. Lentils for lunch and rice pudding for dinner do not provide a complete protein.

When incomplete proteins are combined, not only should foods that supplement limited amino acids be included, they should be combined in proportion to each other for the most efficient utilization of protein. The ratio is specific for each combination. Some examples are:

¾ cup dry rice in combination with ¼ cup dry beans
¾ cup dry rice in combination with 1 cup milk or ¼ cup milk powder

3¼ cups wheat flour in combination with ¼ cup soy grits
and ½ cup sesame seeds

Complementation of proteins is also a practical way to enhance the value of foods readily accepted by young children.
For example, some ways of accomplishing this are by adding
a small amount of soy grits to oatmeal while cooking, or adding wheat germ, soy flour, and dry milk to muffins, pancakes,
and breads.

A simple method, called the Cornell Triple Rich Flour Formula, developed at Cornell University, complements the proteins in baked goods. Before flour is measured, the following
ingredients should go into the bottom of each cup:

1 tbsp. soy flour
1 tbsp. dry milk
1 tsp. wheat germ

Then the flour is added to the desired amount.

As essential as protein is to the body's well-being, it is important to remember that if a child is put on a restricted diet,
such as a vegetarian diet, there is a danger of an inadequate
protein supply. A pure vegetarian (vegan) diet eliminates all
animal foods, thus removing all concentrated sources of protein, calcium, and vitamin B_{12}. A lacto-ovo vegetarian diet
eliminates all meat from the general diet, but includes eggs,
milk, and other dairy products. Some lacto-ovo vegetarian
diets may include fish and occasionally poultry. Based on individual food choices, a lacto-ovo vegetarian diet can be adequate in all nutrients. For the young child, however, it is
difficult to provide sufficient quality and quantity of proteins
in the diet, and an adequate amount of calories and minerals
to support normal growth, using a pure vegetarian (vegan)
diet.

*No extreme diet should be undertaken without first consulting a
doctor and having a complete understanding of what is involved.*

TABLE OF INCOMPLETE PROTEINS		
For quality protein from vegetable sources, use a food from Column I only in combination with a food from Column II.		
	Column I	*Column II*
Legumes	Beans: black-eyed peas, fava, kidney, lima, marrow, mung, navy, peanuts (peanut butter), peas, pinto, snap green beans, soy (tofu)	Dairy products: cheese, cottage cheese, eggs, milk, yogurt Grains Vegetables
Grains	Whole grains: barley, brown rice, buckwheat, bulgur, corn (bread, on the cob, tortillas), grits, oats, rye, wheat germ, whole wheat	Dairy products Legumes Nuts and seeds Vegetables
Vegetables	Asparagus, beet greens, broccoli, Brussels sprouts, cauliflower, chard, collard greens, kale, mustard greens, okra, spinach, sweet potatoes, winter squash, yams	Dairy products Grains Legumes Nuts and seeds Potatoes
Nuts and Seeds	Nuts: almonds, beechnuts, Brazil nuts, cashews, filberts, pecans, pine nuts, walnuts Seeds: pumpkin, sunflower	Dairy products Grains Legumes Vegetables

TABLE OF RECOMMENDED DAILY DIETARY ALLOWANCES FOR PROTEIN, 1989					
	Weight		Height		Energy	Protein
	(kg.)	(lb.)	(cm.)	(in.)	(kcal.)	(g.)
Infants 0.5–1 yr.	9	20	71	28	850	14
Children 1–3 yrs.	13	29	90	35	1,300	16

SOURCE: *Recommended Dietary Allowances*, Food and Nutrition Board, National Academy of Sciences, National Research Council, Washington, D.C. rev. ed. 1989.

NOTE: kg. = kilogram   1 kg. = 2.2 lbs.   1 lb. = .45 kg.
cm. = centimeter 1 cm. = 0.39 inch 1 inch = 2.54 cm.
kcal. = 1,000 calories
g. = gram   1 g. = 0.35 ounce 1 ounce = 28.35g.

FATS

Most of us should cut down on the amount of fat we consume. We do, however, need a certain amount of fat for good health. Fats contain nutritional components called essential fatty acids that are necessary for proper growth and without which we may develop rashes, scaling skin, and hair loss.

Fat is a component of every cell in the body and serves a number of important functions. It acts as a storage depot for energy and other nutrients, is a conductor of heat, and serves very well as insulation against temperature extremes. Our kidneys are protected from injury by the fat that surrounds them.

On a practical level, fats take longer to digest than other

foods, help us feel full, and give certain foods their distinctive tastes and aromas.

Fats also carry the fat-soluble vitamins A, D, E, and K. If we cut out fat in our diets, we also knock out the nutrients that travel with them, and this, carried to extremes, would result in vitamin deficiencies. As there are plenty of meats and vegetables containing fats, a varied diet will prevent this from happening. Some other sources of fat are butter, margarine, vegetable oils, egg yolk, nuts, cheese, mayonnaise, peanut butter, whole milk, and cream.

For health reasons, dietary fats should be kept to a minimum, especially the saturated fats. Food products from land animals generally contain saturated fat, as do a few from vegetable origin, such as coconut and palm kernel oils, which are found in commercial cookies, cake mixes, and nondairy sour cream and whipped toppings. Saturated fats tend to raise the level of cholesterol in the blood and (together with inherited genes) are the villains in arteriosclerosis and heart disease.

Most oils of vegetable origin, such as corn, cottonseed, safflower, sesame, soybean, and sunflower seed, are polyunsaturated and best to use for cooking and in salads.

There are certain monounsaturated fats that do not raise or lower the cholesterol level. These are called neutral fats. Olive oil, peanut oil, peanut butter, avocados, and nuts (except walnuts, which contain polyunsaturated oil) are primarily neutral in their fat content.

Excess fat in the diet is better replaced with carbohydrates such as whole-grain breads and cereals, fruits, vegetables, and potatoes. These foods provide vitamins, minerals, and fiber (nature's laxative) as well as calories.

CHOLESTEROL

Experts in the health and nutrition fields recommend low-fat, low-cholesterol diets for children, with the anticipation of reducing the risk of heart disease later in life.

As the United States has the highest rate of cardiovascular and coronary diseases in the world, and heart disease is the major cause of death in adults, there is just cause for concern here. Studies show that coronary heart disease may start in childhood and progress slowly into adulthood. Although diet is not the only factor in developing heart disease, it is a significant one.

The National Cholesterol Education Program recommends limiting saturated fatty acids to 10 percent of calories, and to limit fat intake to 30 percent of calories and cholesterol intake to 300 milligrams per day. This can be achieved by emphasizing a balanced diet, including more fruits, vegetables, grains, breads, cereals, and legumes, as well as low-fat dairy products, fish, poultry without skin, and moderate amounts of lean red meat in place of foods high in saturated fat.

Although these recommendations are excellent for most of the family, it is very important to understand that *infants under two years of age should not be included in this recommendation*. Babies require more fat in their diets than older children, and cholesterol is essential for babies' growth. In fact, breast milk has more cholesterol in it than whole cow's milk. Babies should not be put on a low-cholesterol diet, and should be given whole milk until the age of two, according to the American Academy of Pediatrics.

CARBOHYDRATES

An increase in the consumption of carbohydrates is now recommended for American families, as they are essential in providing energy as well as being the body's raw fuel. When ingested, some carbohydrates, in the form of glucose, are used for immediate energy needs, some are stored in the liver and muscles, and the remainder are converted to fat. An important function of carbohydrates is to spare proteins from having to supply body energy, leaving them to fulfill the proteins' role in building and repairing body tissue.

Carbohydrates are divided into two groups: *simple carbohydrates* and *complex carbohydrates*. The first group contains sugars and the second contains starches, which also supply bulk and fiber.

The three simple carbohydrates are glucose, fructose, and galactose. Glucose is moderately sweet and, although found in a few foods such as corn syrup, it is chiefly produced in the body by digested starches. All other forms of sugar are converted by the body into glucose. Fructose is found in fruit and honey, and galactose is made in the body by digested lactose (milk sugar).

Carbohydrates also contain "double sugars," the three primary ones being sucrose, lactose, and maltose. Sucrose is common table sugar (large amounts of which have been linked to increased dental cavities in infants and children). It is found in many food sources, including cane and beet sugars, sorghum, molasses, and maple syrup. Small amounts of sucrose occur naturally in most fruits and many vegetables.

Lactose is the sugar found in milk and is the major dietary carbohydrate consumed by infants.

Maltose occurs in malt products and germinated cereals.

The complex carbohydrates include starches, dextrin, cellulose, pectin, and other forms of fiber. Starch is by far the most important of these and accounts for about half the total carbohydrate intake in the American diet. In many other countries starch is the staple food, making up an even higher proportion of the total diet.

Cellulose and other fibers are not digested by the human body, but remain in the digestive tract, contributing important bulk to the diet. This bulk helps move the digested food mass through the system. The main sources of cellulose are stems and leaves of vegetables, seeds, and grain coverings and hulls.

The best food sources for carbohydrates are breads, cereals, flour products, noodles and pasta, grains and rice, potatoes, peas, beans, vegetables, and fruits.

FIBER

Fiber has recently been of great public interest, following indications that it might help prevent certain diseases such as colon cancer, obesity, coronary heart disease, diverticulitis, and irritable bowel syndrome, all of which have been at least partially linked to low-fiber, high-cholesterol, and high-saturated-fat diets.

Fiber is the part of food that resists digestion in the human gastrointestinal tract. It is found only in plants (not in the sinewy parts of meats, as is sometimes believed).

There are two different terms used in reference to fiber: *crude fiber* and *dietary fiber*. This can cause confusion when trying to estimate the amount of fiber contained in a specific product, but the fiber content listed on packages usually refers to crude fiber. *Crude fiber* is the food material (consisting primarily of cellulose) that remains after the food has gone through the digestive process.

Dietary fiber includes more substances than crude fiber. It is a mixture of complex carbohydrates that are largely resistant to human digestion, such as cellulose, hemicellulose, pectin, and a non-carbohydrate called lignin.* Crude-fiber analysis does not accurately reflect the entire amount of dietary fiber in food products. It apparently represents only one fifth to one half the total dietary fiber present in food.

Although the physiological effects of dietary fiber are not completely understood, increased amounts of fiber in the diet result in decreased intestinal transit time, increased stool-water content, and, in certain circumstances, a reduction in cholesterol.

Unfortunately, most of the research performed on the benefits of fiber relates to adults. Now the important question is, should fiber in the diet of infants, toddlers, and children be increased? If so, this would necessitate an increase in the consumption of fruits, vegetables, legumes, and whole-grain ce-

*Pectin is, however, one fiber substance that is digested.

reals and breads. A recent study showed that a large percentage of children eat less than the recommended daily amounts of fruits and vegetables, breads, and cereals. This would indicate that there *is* a need for children to increase their intake of fiber-containing foods.

However, some objections have been made to increasing fiber in a child's diet. One reason is that a child has a limited stomach capacity. High-fiber foods are low in calories but high in bulk, thereby diminishing the child's ability to receive an adequate caloric intake. Another objection is that dietary fiber may adversely influence the absorption of certain essential minerals, such as calcium, iron, copper, magnesium, phosphorus, and zinc. The American Academy of Pediatrics feels that a substantial amount of fiber should probably be consumed to ensure normal laxation.

It seems unlikely that fiber is necessary for babies less than twelve months old, but with the introduction of solid foods into the diets of older children, care should be taken to include whole-grain breads, cereals, fruits, and vegetables. However, a diet that places emphasis on high-fiber, low-calorie foods, to the exclusion of the other common food groups, would not be recommended for children.

The table on pages 32–33 shows the fiber content of common foods, as well as portions that should be served to one- to three-year-olds.

VITAMINS

The word "vitamin" means living substance. Vitamins are organic compounds, essential for proper utilization of food and healthy functioning of the body. They have been referred to as invisible helpers, ready to aid in building and maintaining a perfect body. However, the body cannot manufac-

FIBER CONTENT OF FOODS (per 100 mg)*		
Food	Little Fiber (0.2 gm)	Low Fiber (0.5 gm; range 0.3–1 gm)
Bread	Cracked wheat, white, rye, pumpernickel breads; white crackers	Whole wheat bread and crackers
Cereals	Rice, macaroni, noodles, spaghetti	Barley, brown rice, Cheerios, cornflakes, farina, oatmeal, puffed rice, shredded wheat, Wheaties
Vegetables		Asparagus, beets, cabbage, carrots, celery, collards, corn, cucumbers, eggplant, lettuce, mushrooms, onions, sweet potato, white potato with or without skin, spinach, summer squash, tomato, white turnip
Fruits	Juices only	Applesauce, apricots, banana, canned fruit cocktail, cherries, grapefruit, grapes, mango, melon, oranges, papaya, pears without skin, pineapple, plums, prunes, raisins, rhubarb

SOURCE: *Diet Manual Massachusetts General Hospital*, Little, Brown, Boston, 1976.

Moderate Fiber (1.5 gm; range 1.1–2.0 gm)	High Fiber (3 gm; range 2.1–4.2 gm)	Serving size for 1–3 yrs.
		½ slice of bread 4 servings
40% bran flakes, puffed wheat, raisin bran	All-Bran (4.8 gm/ cup), wheat germ (2.5 gm/cup)	½ oz (½ cup) ready-to-eat cereal; ¼ cup cooked cereal or pasta 4 servings
Green and wax beans, dried beans and peas (kidney, lentils, lima, soybeans, split pea, etc.), broccoli, Brussels sprouts, cauliflower, dandelion, kale, mustard greens, fresh or frozen green peas, okra, parsnip, peppers, pumpkin, rutabaga, winter squash	Artichoke, 1 large (2.4 gm), green peas, canned only (2.3 gm/½ cup)	¼ cup 2 servings or more
Apples, avocado, berries (except blackberries), figs, fresh pears with skin	Fresh blackberries (4.1 gm/¾ cup), dried dates (2.3 gm/ ½ cup), dried figs (5.6 gm/cup)	¼ cup fruit; ¼ cup juice 2 servings or more; fruits with pits not advised

*Fiber values assigned are based on data in *Composition of Foods—Raw, Processed, Prepared* (Agricultural Handbook No. 8), Bernice K. Watt, and Annabel L. Merrill, U.S. Department of Agriculture, Agricultural Research Service, Washington, D.C., 1963.

ture vitamins with the exception of vitamin K, so it must receive them through food, drink, and sun. Each vitamin performs a special function and, although only small quantities are required, a serious deficiency of any one could prove disastrous. A well-balanced diet will supply adequate amounts of all the vitamins.

Vitamin pills are not intended to be, and should not be used as, a substitute for vitamin foods. However, if a child's appetite is poor or his eating habits so bad that he is not getting a balanced diet, fat-soluble and water-soluble vitamins may be added. But remember that vitamins cannot compensate for a diet lacking in fats, proteins, and carbohydrates, and that too many vitamins can be as dangerous as too few. Also, fat-soluble vitamins are stored in the body, so excessive quantities may eventually produce toxic effects.

VITAMINS AND/OR MINERALS SHOULD NOT BE GIVEN WITHOUT FIRST CONSULTING YOUR DOCTOR.

The fat-soluble vitamins are A, D, E, and K, and the water-soluble vitamins are the B complex group and C. Fat-soluble vitamins can be stored by the body for later use, but unused water-soluble vitamins are excreted in the urine. Foods containing the water-soluble vitamins must be eaten daily in order to supply the body constantly.

VITAMIN A helps keep the skin healthy and protects it from becoming rough and dry. An insufficiency of this vitamin can cause nails to split or become ridged, and hair will lose its luster and grow dry and brittle. It is important for growth, strong bones, and healthy teeth in children. The linings of the gastrointestinal and respiratory tracts require vitamin A to function properly. It also helps build resistance to infection. Vitamin A is necessary for good vision and protects against night blindness.

Symptoms of vitamin A deficiency are night blindness, stunted growth, tooth and gum decay, loss of appetite, dry or scaly skin, loss of vigor, sinus trouble, and increased susceptibility to infection. However, vitamin A deficiency is rare in this country, and toxicity caused by taking excessive amounts does occur.

Best food sources for vitamin A are liver, fish liver oils, butter, milk, and egg yolk.

Beta carotene is a provitamin from which the body manufactures vitamin A. Extensive research is ongoing on the beneficial effect of beta carotene in preventing lung cancer and possibly other cancers. Beta carotene cannot be taken in vitamin A pills, but must be ingested through fruits and vegetables containing this substance.

Sources rich in carotene are sweet potatoes, carrots, collard greens, beet greens, spinach, pumpkin, butternut squash, tomatoes, broccoli, red peppers, winter squash, cantaloupe, apricots, papayas, peaches, and nectarines.

The vitamin B complex group contains eight water-soluble vitamins: B_1 (thiamine), B_2 (riboflavin), B_6 (pyridoxine), B_{12} (cyanocobalamin), niacin, folic acid, pantothenic acid, and biotin.

VITAMIN B_1 (thiamine) is necessary for growth, good appetite and digestion, and healthy nerves. It helps the body release food-supplied energy.

Best food sources are pork, organ meats, whole grains, brewer's yeast, eggs, and cereals.

VITAMIN B_2 (riboflavin) helps blood cells utilize oxygen. It also assists in maintaining good vision and is needed in certain enzymes that help change food into energy. Important for smooth skin, it is beneficial in preventing scaling or cracking of skin around the mouth and nose.

Good sources are liver, milk and milk products, green leafy vegetables, meats, eggs, and whole-grain and enriched bread's and cereals.

VITAMIN B_6 (pyridoxine) is necessary for growth and a healthy nervous system.

Best food sources are organ meats, pork, bran, and wheat germ.

VITAMIN B$_{12}$ (cyanocobalamin) is involved in many processes necessary to metabolize proteins, fats, and carbohydrates. It also participates in the formation of red blood cells. Deficiency of this vitamin is uncommon except in children who have been put on a vegan diet (no animal protein, milk, eggs, or cheese).

Symptoms of deficiency include tiredness, breathlessness, sore tongue, nervous lesions, and megaloblastic anemia. Serious deficiency may cause irreversible neurological damage unless diagnosed and treated early.

Vitamin B$_{12}$ occurs only in animal foods. Lean meats, liver, kidney, eggs, and fish are all excellent sources. Vitamin B$_{12}$ is also found in milk and cheese.

NIACIN promotes normal appetite and digestion and is necessary for a healthy nervous system. It is also needed in certain enzymes that help convert food into energy.

Good sources of niacin are liver, meats, fish, poultry, green vegetables, nuts (especially peanuts), whole-grain breads and cereals (except corn), and enriched breads and cereals.

FOLIC ACID (folacin) is important for proper development of red blood cells.

Best food sources are green leafy vegetables, liver, beef, yeast, and orange juice.

PANTOTHENIC ACID aids in metabolism and the synthesis of adrenal hormones.

Best food sources are eggs, liver, and salmon. However, all animal and plant foods contain certain amounts of pantothenic acid.

BIOTIN assists in metabolism of proteins, carbohydrates, and fats.

Best food sources are liver, peanuts, milk, meats, most vegetables, egg yolk, brewer's yeast, and brown rice.

VITAMIN C (ascorbic acid) has many functions. It helps the gastrointestinal absorption of iron and calcium, protects vita-

mins A and E, and is necessary for formation of certain substances that cement bone cells, teeth, connective tissue, and
capillaries. Vitamin C provides resistance to disease and aids
in healing wounds.

VITAMIN TABLE*						
	Water-Soluble Vitamins					
	Vit. B_1 (mg)	Vit. B_2 (mg)	Vit. B_6 (mg)	Vit. B_{12} (μg)	Niacin (mg)	Folic Acid (μg)	Vit. C (mg)
Infants 0.5–1 yr.	0.4	0.5	0.6	0.5	6	35	35
Children 1–3 yrs.	0.7	0.8	1.0	0.7	9	50	40

Fat-Soluble Vitamins				
	Vit. A (μg RE)	Vit. D (μg)	Vit. E (mg)	Vit. K (μg)
Infants 0.5–1 yr.	375	10	4	10
Children 1–3 yrs.	400	10	6	15

Note: RE = retinal equivalent
Legend: g = gram   1 g = .035 ounce   1 ounce = 28.35 g
mg = milligram, one thousandth of a gram
μg = microgram, one millionth of a gram

*Source: *Recommended Dietary Allowances*, Revised 1989, Food and Nutrition Board, National Academy of Sciences, National Research Council, Washington, D.C.

Vitamin C should be replenished daily. It is lost rapidly
when kept at room temperature, but much less so when refrigerated. Frozen foods should not be thawed before cooking,
as this causes a great loss of vitamin C. Vegetables should be
either steamed or cooked in a tightly covered pan with a small

amount of liquid, over a low heat. Soda should never be used in cooking vegetables, as it destroys vitamin C.

Vitamin C deficiency causes scurvy (symptoms are tender, painful muscles, joints, and bones, muscle cramps, and loss of appetite) and gum disease.

Best vegetable sources are broccoli, Brussels sprouts, cabbage, cauliflower, spinach, red and green peppers, tomatoes, and potatoes.

Best fruit sources for vitamin C are cantaloupe, grapefruit, oranges, limes, lemons, strawberries, tangerines, kiwi fruit, and watermelon.

VITAMIN D is important in building strong bones and teeth. A daily supply is necessary for the body to use calcium from food and to release calcium stored in the bones. Some vitamin D can be produced by the body through the action of direct sunlight on the skin. If sunshine is not available, a dietary source of vitamin D is essential.

Best food source is fish liver oils. However, these are seldom included in most diets because of the taste, and children refuse them. Other sources are vitamin D fortified milk, egg yolk, and liver.

VITAMIN E prevents destruction of certain other nutrients (vitamin A) in the body and aids in the proper use of energy supplied by glucose and fatty acids. It is also necessary for healthy red blood cells.

This vitamin is found primarily in foods of plant origin, such as vegetable oils, wheat germ, nuts, whole-grain breads and cereals, and dark green leafy vegetables.

VITAMIN K is necessary for normal clotting of blood. Dietary requirements for this vitamin are normally quite low because it is formed in the intestine.

Vitamin K sources are found in a variety of vegetables such as cabbage, cauliflower, spinach, Swiss chard, and beet greens.

MINERALS

Minerals are needed for our health and well-being. They have two general functions, to build and regulate the body. Each mineral has a special activity which is of equal importance to the others. The building function affects the skeleton and all soft tissue, and the regulation function involves a wide variety of systems such as heartbeat, blood clotting, maintenance of the internal pressure of body fluids, nerve responses, and transportation of oxygen from the lungs to the tissues.

Some of these functions require large quantities of minerals, while others may need only minute traces. Without minerals, the vitamins cannot perfect their work. However, minerals can be harmful if taken in excess, and each year many children under five years of age are hospitalized with iron poisoning caused by accidentally swallowing multiple vitamin and mineral supplements. A balanced diet usually supplies all the minerals the body needs.

In cooking vegetables and grains, it is essential that excessive heat be avoided, that a minimum of water be used, and that airtight lids cover saucepans to prevent oxidation in order to retain maximum nutrients and avoid loss of precious minerals.

Minerals found in the human body fall into two groups: *major minerals*, if present in large amounts; and *trace minerals*, if present in small amounts and with a known function, or if present in small amounts with a function that is not understood.

Major minerals are calcium, phosphorus, magnesium, sodium, chloride, and potassium.

Trace minerals are iron, zinc, iodine, selenium, copper, manganese, fluoride, chromium, and molybdenum.

Of all the minerals listed above, calcium, potassium, phosphorus, magnesium, copper, zinc, fluoride, iodine, and iron will be dealt with here in more detail.

CALCIUM is the mineral found in the body in the largest quantity. It is essential for the formation of strong bones and teeth. Although 99 percent of the body's calcium is in the bones and teeth, the remaining 1 percent is in the blood, body fluids, and soft tissues, where it plays a very important role.

Calcium is required for proper blood clotting, transmission of nerve impulses, and contraction and relaxation of the heart. These functions are so important that the body will extract calcium from the bones if necessary.

Growing children need large amounts of calcium. The daily requirement for infants six months to one year is 600 milligrams, and for children one to three years it is 800 milligrams. A healthy person normally absorbs 20 to 30 percent of the calcium ingested. If the need for calcium should increase, so

CALCIUM CONTENT OF SOME COMMON FOODS		
Food	*Amount*	*Calcium (mg)*
Plain yogurt	1 cup	425
Fruit and flavored yogurt	1 cup	380
Sardines with bones	3 oz.	360
Milk (whole, low-fat, nonfat, buttermilk, chocolate)	1 cup	300
Swiss and Gruyère cheeses	1 oz.	270
Hard cheeses (Cheddar, Monterey Jack, Edam, Muenster)	1 oz.	200
Processed cheeses	1 oz.	175
Salmon with bones	3 oz.	170
Collard greens	½ cup	170
Cheese spreads	1 oz.	160
Soft cheeses (mozzarella, blue, feta)	1 oz.	150
Cheese foods	1 oz.	140
Turnip greens, kale, dandelion greens	½ cup	100
Cooked dried beans (navy, pea, and lima)	1 cup	90

does its absorption by the body, and growing children may absorb up to 75 percent of the calcium they consume.

Calcium absorption is promoted by the presence of lactose, vitamin D, and the parathyroid hormone, while a dietary excess of phosphorus will hinder calcium absorption. Many commercial soft drinks, and especially colas, contain phosphoric acid.

The best food sources of calcium are milk and dairy products, sardines and salmon with bones, dark green leafy vegetables (except spinach), and dried beans.

POTASSIUM acts in balance with sodium as a major control for water distribution in the body. It is about twice as plentiful in the body as sodium. The average diet contains an ample supply of potassium, so a deficiency is unlikely. This mineral is widely distributed in natural foods such as legumes, whole grains, green leafy vegetables, and meats, and in certain fruits such as bananas, dates, oranges, and dried prunes.

PHOSPHORUS. Eighty percent of the body's phosphorus is found in the bones. The remaining 20 percent is contained in muscle and blood serum. Phosphorus is a necessary constituent of every cell in the body.

Recommended intakes of phosphorus are the same as for calcium, except during infancy, when a dietary calcium-to-phosphorus ratio of 1.5 to 1 is recommended. Phosphorus is found along with calcium in dairy products, but it also exists in foods containing little calcium, including such protein-rich foods as meats, eggs, nuts, and legumes. It is also found in grains and is present in many carbonated beverages.

MAGNESIUM is the fourth most abundant mineral in the body; approximately 50 percent of it is found in the bones, along with calcium and phosphorus, 25 percent in the muscles, and the remainder in soft tissue. It is necessary for the production and transfer of energy and helps conduct the nerve impulses that relax muscles following contraction. Magnesium also seems to promote calcium retention in tooth enamel and increase resistance to dental cavities.

Magnesium is relatively widespread in nature. Nuts, whole grains, soybeans, legumes, and shellfish are excellent sources. It exists in all green plants as a component of chlorophyll.

COPPER. Trace amounts of copper are distributed in all tissues throughout the body. The highest concentration of this mineral is found in the liver, brain, and kidneys. One of copper's most important functions is to facilitate the absorption and transportation of iron throughout the body.

The requirement for copper is so low, and it appears in so many foods, that deficiencies are unlikely to occur in normal children who consume a variety of foods.

The richest sources of copper are shellfish, organ meats, dried legumes, eggs, and nuts. Substantial quantities of copper may be present in drinking water supplied through copper pipes, especially in soft-water areas.

ZINC. The biological role of zinc has been recognized for more than a hundred years, but only recently has its importance attracted attention in nutrition. The human body contains only about 2 grams of zinc, yet this mineral is absolutely essential for proper growth and development and for normal body functioning.

Zinc plays diverse roles in everyday life. It is vital for the health of the skin, the healing of wounds, and maintaining a normal sense of taste. It is a component of many enzymes involved in metabolism, and it is essential for the formation of the nucleic acids RNA and DNA, the basic materials of genes. Zinc enhances the action of a number of hormones, including insulin, and is essential for normal growth and development of the embryo and newborn infant. The possibility of zinc deficiency should be considered in any child with poor appetite and slow growth. Recommended daily dietary allowance of zinc for children six months to one year is 5 milligrams, and for children one to three years of age, 10 milligrams.

Zinc-rich foods include organ meats (2 ounces of liver contain about 4 milligrams of zinc), muscle meats (the dark meat of poultry is a particularly good source, with 3 ounces providing 2.4 milligrams), dairy products (a cup of milk contains 1 milligram), and eggs (one egg contains 0.5 milligram). Whole-grain cereals are high in zinc, but they also contain substances called phytates that combine with the mineral and interfere with absorption. However, when whole grains are sprouted or used in making bread with yeast, the phytates are inactivated, allowing for more efficient absorption. Like most trace minerals, much of the zinc is removed when grains are processed, so breads and cereals made from refined flours are generally a poor source. The key to getting enough zinc is to have a diet containing plenty of fresh and minimally processed foods, in addition to the high-zinc food sources.

FLUORIDE. This essential element is present in varying concentrations in practically all soils, water supplies, plants, and animals, as well as in the blood, bones, and teeth of the human body.

The National Academy of Sciences has classified fluoride as a beneficial trace element because of its value to the maintenance of healthy teeth. From conception, fluoride is needed for the formation of teeth; after birth it is necessary for the maintenance of healthy bones and teeth, once both primary and permanent teeth have emerged. Fluoride strengthens enamel, making it more resistant to tooth decay, can contribute to the growth of new enamel in early decay, and has the ability to destroy some bacteria that convert sugar to acids in the mouth.

Research shows that proper use of fluoride can reduce dental decay by 40 to 60 percent when used from birth throughout adulthood. Consequently, dental decay among schoolchildren is lower now than ever before, and increasing numbers of adults are retaining their teeth throughout their lives.

As with other essential elements, such as iron, vitamins A and D, and oxygen, which are also necessary for the body's life and good health, fluoride can be toxic in excessive quantities. Its safety range, however, is very wide, and large amounts of fluoride would have to be ingested over an extended period of time to present a significant health problem. Early indications of excessive intake of fluoride are recognized by either a slight discoloration, or white spots, on the permanent teeth.

Fluoride is administered to children in two very distinct ways: systemically and topically. Systemic application simply means that fluoride drops are given orally to babies, or in tablet form to older children during the time teeth and bones are being formed. Although permanent teeth do not start to erupt until around the fifth birthday, enamel begins to form at birth, and the process continues until around the thirteenth year.

Topical application of fluoride is given to already formed tooth enamel by mouth rinse, toothpaste, topical gel in dental offices, or in what is known as a "swish-wash" mouth-rinse program, which is administered by elementary schools in unfluoridated water areas. All of these methods prove effective in preventing tooth decay and do not affect the development of teeth and bones. Topically applied fluoride is not meant to be swallowed, although studies show that children do swallow most of the toothpaste they use from the time they start brushing until around their seventh birthday. This may increase the total fluoride intake beyond the recommended daily dosage.

Once your toddler starts brushing, it is important that he be supervised to ensure that only a small quantity of toothpaste is put on the brush and that the toothpaste is not swallowed. However, always encourage brushing *after* meals.

Parents, along with the child's dentist and pediatrician, should be fully aware of how much fluoride a child is receiving. Factors to consider are: age, weight, fluoride content in local water supplies, amount of water consumed through prepared formula or baby foods, whether the baby is receiving only breast milk with no added water through supplements, and, once the child starts brushing, how much toothpaste is being swallowed.

Whether you are breast-feeding or have your baby on formula or cow's milk will also affect your little one's daily fluoride intake. Breast and cow's milk are naturally low in fluoride, containing approximately 0.1 ppm (parts per million). Premixed formula contains 0.3 ppm. The amount of fluoride in dry or concentrated formula will depend on the fluoride level in your local water supply, a number that can be established through your local health or water department.

The optimal use of fluoride involves a delicate balance between the protection against dental cavities and the avoidance of dental fluorosis.

As confirmed in a 1991 report by the U.S. Public Health Service, "Fluoride has substantial benefits in the prevention of dental caries," and virtually all major health organizations* endorse and support the use of fluoride as an important tool in promoting dental health.

IODINE. The largest amount of iodine in the body is focused in the thyroid gland, and small amounts are present in the blood, skin, and other tissues. The thyroid hormones regulate energy metabolism. The conversion of carotene to vitamin A, the synthesis of proteins, and the intestinal absorption of carbohydrates are more efficient when thyroid hormone levels are normal.

The recommended daily requirement of iodine for infants six months to one year is 50 micrograms (a microgram is one millionth of a gram), and for children one to three, 70 micrograms.

Iodized salt, milk, and seafood are the best sources of dietary iodine. The fact that the iodine content of food is determined by the soil in which the food is grown is no longer significant in the etiology of iodine deficiency. Food that is consumed in one area is often transported from another. It has also become a practice to enrich animal feeds with iodine in places where the soil is deficient in it.

IRON is the most abundant trace mineral in the body. It is necessary for the formation of hemoglobin, which carries oxygen to the body's cells and carbon dioxide away from the tis-

*The American Academy of Pediatrics, the American Dental Association, U.S. Public Health Service, Department of Health Education & Welfare, the Environmental Protection Agency, the Food & Drug Administration, the American Heart Association, the National Cancer Institute, the Pharmaceutical Association, and the World Health Organization.

sues. The recommended daily allowance for children six months to three years is 10 milligrams.

IRON CONTENT OF SOME COMMON FOODS		
Food	*Amount*	*Iron (mg)*
Iron-fortified formula	8 oz.	3.0
Infant cereal, high protein	1 tbsp.	1.1
Infant cereal, rice	1 tbsp.	1.1
Strained beef with vegetables	1 oz.	0.3
Strained split peas with ham	1 oz.	0.2
Strained vegetables and chicken	1 oz.	0.1
Strained beef	1 oz.	0.6
Strained liver	1 oz.	1.6
Hamburger, cooked	2 oz.	1.8
Chicken, dark meat	1 oz.	0.5
Beef liver	1 oz.	2.5
Chicken liver	1 liver	2.1
Liverwurst	1 oz.	1.7
Frankfurter	1	0.9
Egg	1 medium	1.0
Pork and beans	¼ cup	1.5
Peanut butter	1 tbsp.	0.3
Bread, enriched white	1 slice	0.7
Macaroni, enriched, cooked	¼ cup	0.4
Carrots, cooked	¼ cup	0.2
Orange	1 medium	0.6
Canned pears	¼ cup	0.1

Although there may be a large intake of iron, intestinal absorption may vary. Different types of iron also affect absorption. Only approximately 10 percent of the iron taken in by infants and children is absorbed.

Once an infant starts on solids, the best source of iron is iron-fortified baby cereal. Few commercially prepared baby foods provide generous amounts of iron, with the exception of pure beef and liver. Organ meats, dried legumes, shellfish, and muscle meats provide the richest and most usable sources of iron. Other sources include nuts, green leafy vegetables, and whole wheat flour and bread.

MINERAL TABLE*					
	Calcium (mg)	*Phosphorus (mg)*	*Magnesium (mg)*	*Zinc (mg)*	*Iodine (μg)*	*Iron (mg)*
Infants 0.5–1 yr.	600	500	60	5	50	10
Children 1–3 yrs.	800	800	80	10	70	10

Legend: μg = microgram (one millionth of a gram)
mg = milligram (one thousandth of a gram)
g = gram

Iron deficiency anemia is still a major problem among infants and young children.

Four factors determine adequate iron supplies in infants and children:

• Iron endowment at birth
• Relative growth rate
• Occult-blood loss
• Iron intake and absorption

*Source: *Recommended Dietary Allowances*, Revised 1989, Food and Nutrition Board, National Academy of Sciences, National Research Council, Washington, D.C.

Feeding Children

FEEDING children well can be a challenge to any parent. In many homes, a child's eating habits and mealtime behavior are sources of great stress for both parents and child. Parents who adopt a relaxed attitude toward food and mealtimes are more successful in getting their children to eat nutritious, well-balanced meals. However, any child's appetite can fluctuate from month to month, especially while he goes through the teething process for the first two years or so.

Mealtimes should be and can be enjoyable for parents and baby, although it may occasionally take a conscious effort to make them so. There is no way of getting around the fact that a baby learning to eat solid foods creates a mess. After every meal during this stage, the child, high chair, floor, and often parent have to be washed. If you can remember that this stage doesn't last forever and learn to be prepared, it can be fun.

It is to every child's advantage to be exposed to a wide variety of foods, although they do not need those that are highly seasoned. It is fine to introduce Mexican, Indian, or other ethnic dishes with various herbs and spices, but the flavors should be mild. Children prefer the natural taste of foods, and salt can be eliminated in most cooking.

What a child eats is much more important than how much

he eats. Parental buying habits can do much to diminish the problems of bad eating habits. If nonnutritive foods are not in your home in the first place, they cannot be consumed by the child. If a child is not exposed to cookies, candies, and other sweets, he is not going to insist on them in place of vegetables, fruit, cheese, or meat.

Parents may not be aware of how little food a child needs, especially when he is switched from baby to table food. Infants cannot eat and do not need adult-size portions. The age at which many children begin eating table food (twelve months to two years) coincides with the age at which their growth rate and appetite naturally decrease. As a guideline: *The average child can be expected to eat one tablespoonful of each type of food at each meal for each year of his age.*

From about one and a half years on, the child starts to be demanding and fussy and can be adamant about what he wants and doesn't want. Coaxing or persuasion seldom helps. That is why establishing the child's taste for nutritious, wholesome foods from the very beginning is so important. His tastes are going to change, and some of the foods he accepted earlier are likely to be flatly refused now. But a child's basic food preferences are going to remain unless parents unknowingly change them.

Children are usually notoriously reluctant to eat vegetables. It seems to me that the way they are served and how frequently have a lot to do with this reaction. Vegetables served freshly steamed or microwaved look and taste so much better than puréed spinach or peas and carrots from a jar. Homemade soups made with a milk base, fresh vegetables, and small pieces of meat and/or rice and beans can ensure that a baby gets his vegetables, even a complete meal, that can be taken from a cup.

Children usually enjoy fruits, so offer them for desserts instead of cookies, cakes, and Jell-O. Dried fruits are wonderful finger foods, and are readily accepted by children in place of candy. Dried pitted dates, prunes, and apricots are also good sources of vitamins and minerals.

Don't fill up your child with snacks such as potato chips and cookies. If an hour or two after eating a substantial meal he appears hungry, offer fruit, cheese, vegetable sticks or chunks, yogurt, a piece of whole wheat bread, rice or wheat cracker, a bagel, a cup of milk, or a fruit or milk drink.

Be sensitive to your little one's own signs telling you what he wants and how he feels, and don't project your desires, decisions, or fears onto your baby. Feed him only when he is hungry. Be relaxed and unconcerned if he refuses food for one or two meals. Here we are talking about healthy babies. However, if you suspect that your child may be sick, you should consult a physician.

Last, let your baby feed himself as soon as he is able, regardless of the mess. Make the atmosphere happy, with smiles, laughter, music if you like, and love.

MILK

Because of its high nutritional value, milk is important to our diet. According to the U.S. Department of Agriculture, dairy products (excluding butter) contribute only 11 percent of food energy (calories), but provide 75 percent of the calcium, 39 percent of the riboflavin, 35 percent of the phosphorus, 22 percent of the magnesium, 20 percent of the vitamin B_{12}, and substantial quantities of other nutrients necessary to a healthful diet.

The American Academy of Pediatrics has recommended that infants not be given whole cow's milk prior to six months of age, but be either breast-fed or receive iron-fortified formulas. (Ideally, it is best not to use cow's milk until your baby reaches his first birthday.) If large amounts of whole milk (one quart or more per day) are consumed without benefit of supplemental iron, serious iron deficiencies may occur. As milk is low in iron, such large quantities would replace the iron-rich foods that should be part of a whole-milk diet.

With the current emphasis on diets lower in fat and cholesterol, mothers may feel inclined to give their infants or toddlers skim or low-fat milk. Fat-reduced milk should not be given to children under two years of age, as it will deprive them of necessary calories and reduce their intake of fats and fatty acids. Diets of normal infants and toddlers should not be restricted this way.

Many Hispanic, Native American, Oriental, and black children suffer from lactose intolerance, a condition in which there is an inability to digest lactose (milk sugar) because of a deficiency of the enzyme lactose. Some symptoms of this condition may be diarrhea, flatulence (gas), abdominal cramps, and bloating. However, the use of milk and milk products should not be discouraged completely, as lactose intolerance to as much as a cup of milk consumed at one time is rare in preadolescents. (Additional sources of calcium are sardines, salmon with bones, turnip greens, and cooked dried beans, among others, but a toddler would not receive an adequate supply from these sources because he would have to eat such large quantities to do so.)

As well as being a good source of protein, calcium, and other valuable nutrients, milk also is sold fortified with vitamin D. The lactose and vitamin D in milk aid in calcium absorption.

EGGS

In addition to being a great source of protein, eggs contain iron (in the yolk) and vitamins A, B, and D, and are therefore a useful food for babies.

Eggs do, however, present two potential health hazards. First, they are high in cholesterol, although the egg industry has managed to reduce the cholesterol level per egg from 274 mg. to approximately 213 mg. Accordingly, the American Heart Association has raised its allowance of eggs for healthy adults, children, and babies from three to four per week.

To reduce the amount of cholesterol consumed, egg white may easily be substituted for whole egg, especially in recipes calling for several eggs.

The second potential problem concerns the possibility of salmonella contamination, which appears to be an increasing problem in eggs. Because of this, raw eggs should not be given in any form to infants or toddlers; their immune systems may not be strong enough to handle any contamination. Here is a list of some standard foods that may contain raw unpasteurized eggs: milk shakes, homemade mayonnaise and ice cream, Caesar salad, Hollandaise sauce, and sunny-side-up eggs, in which the yolk is barely cooked. Soft-boiled eggs are safe if cooked for five minutes in boiling water. Most commercial foods are prepared with pasteurized and sterilized eggs, and are therefore safe.

Eggs may be prepared in many ways in a microwave oven, but will explode if not removed from the shell. Always pierce the egg yolk with a toothpick or fork before poaching. You will discover that scrambled eggs and omelets turn out well when microwaved.

SALT

Sodium, a component of salt or sodium chloride, is one of the more plentiful major minerals in the body and is critical to many metabolic activities. It controls the volume of body fluids and water balance, helps relax contracted muscles (in the presence of potassium), facilitates the absorption of various nutrients, including glucose, and transmits nerve impulses.

Throughout the ages, salt has been considered a precious mineral, and used as one of the world's principal trading commodities. During the late eighteenth century, the rank of guests at a banquet was gauged by where they sat in relation to an elaborate silver saltcellar on the table. The host and distinguished guests sat at the head of the table, above the salt. Those who sat below the salt, farthest from the host, were of little consequence. Today that etiquette could work in reverse.

What has caused a mineral that was once so valued to become our dietary Enemy Number One? Basically most foods contain some sodium, including our drinking water. Salt is used in cooking, then it is added again at the table. We now have an abundance of salt and use a great deal more than we need, feeling that our meals taste bland without it.

Salt, of course, is a taste that one becomes accustomed to. Babies are born with pure taste buds and no bad eating habits, and these can be avoided if they are given unadulterated foods. Eating patterns formed early will stay with a child for the rest of his life.

Statistically it has been shown that there are excessive incidences of hypertension (high blood pressure) in countries where there is a high intake of salt, and hypertension is one of the major health problems of North America. Both hereditary and environmental factors are involved. Studies have shown that children are at greater risk when there is a family history of hypertension. Among environmental factors, salt in the diet has been cited as a possible contributing element. Although there is no definite proof that some humans are particularly sensitive to high salt intake, animal studies have raised that speculation. With individuals potentially at risk, a high salt intake at infancy might predispose them to developing hypertension later in life.

The American Dietetic Association suggests that salt should not be added to homemade baby foods, nor should infants be given canned products containing added salt. The study revealed that milk and milk products alone provide enough sodium to meet the recommended salt intake level for children up to eighteen months of age. It was also found that sodium intake from homemade foods was relatively low during the first six months of life, with a marked increase from six to eight months, and a sharp increase from eight months onward. This was attributed to the use of table foods, which were introduced at the average age of seven months. Eleven percent or less of a baby's total sodium intake before six months was contributed by home-prepared foods. A rapid increase to 52 percent, 60 percent, 72 percent, and 77 percent was noted at ten, twelve, fifteen, and eighteen months of age, respectively.

To give some indication of how much salt is present in certain foods, corn has only 1 milligram; cornflakes have 256 milligrams per cup; a potato has 5 milligrams; ten potato chips have 200 milligrams; a frozen meat-loaf dinner has 1,305 milligrams; a cup of canned tomato soup has 932 milligrams; and a fast-food chicken dinner contains 2,243 milligrams of salt. The estimated safe and adequate daily dietary allowance of sodium for a six- to eleven-month-old is 200 milligrams. For a one-year-old it is 225 milligrams, and for a two- to five-year-old, 300 milligrams a day.*

(The relationship between sodium and salt may be confusing. Salt is composed of two elements, sodium and chloride. Each molecule of salt is 40 percent sodium. One level teaspoon of salt weighing 7 grams contains 2.8 grams, or 2,800 milligrams, of sodium.)

I have always been very conscious of adding little or no salt or sugar to my baby's food, and never use salt when boiling potatoes, macaroni, vegetables, or spaghetti. Occasionally I add a little salt to a recipe, but prefer to add other herbs, spices, and flavors to enhance the food. I feel all of this is beneficial to my whole family's well-being. Although I have not specified it in all applicable recipes, I believe it is wise and preferable to use unsalted (sweet) butter.

SUGAR

The subject of sugar is as controversial as that of salt. Sugar has virtually no nutritional value, destroys the appetite, promotes tooth decay, and is otherwise known as "empty calo-

*1,000 milligrams = 1 gram

ries." As with salt, most foods contain some form of sugar.

The food industry uses sugar liberally as a preservative as well as to sweeten such foods as cakes, cookies, and cereals, some of which are more than 50 percent sugar! Many foods that do not appear to be sweet, such as catsup, bread, canned corn, and mustard, also contain sugar. To avoid an excess of sugar in the diet, it is important to read food labels when shopping, remembering that ingredients are listed in order of quantity.

Some people feel that turbinado sugar, which is partially refined, is more nutritious than white sugar. However, studies by Krehl and Cowgill at Yale University School of Medicine concluded that raw sugar and other sugar products, including brown sugar, contain such small quantities of vitamins as to be insignificant. However, the darkest brown sugar available does contain small amounts of calcium, phosphorus, iron, sodium, and potassium. Blackstrap molasses, perhaps the most "beneficial" of the sweeteners, contains the B complex vitamins, iron, calcium, copper, magnesium, potassium, and phosphorus, as well as being 50 percent natural sugar.

Honey is easily assimilated and is therefore more digestible, but should not be given to babies under one year as it may contain botulism spores. Recent data show that there has been a significant increase in infant botulism in babies under a year who have been fed honey. While older children and adults can consume honey that may contain botulism spores without experiencing any problems, infants have no protective mechanisms to defeat the organism, as their intestines are still undeveloped.

Chocolate is another controversial sweet that contains empty calories. It also contains caffeine, theobromine, and oxalic acid, which are not recommended for babies. Carob—high in iron, minerals, calcium, and vitamins, and low in fat—can be substituted for chocolate. However, it is suggested that all sweets and sweeteners be given extremely sparingly to young children to prevent the encouragement of a sweet tooth.

NURSING BOTTLE SYNDROME AND YOUR BABY'S TEETH

Bottle feeding is one method of giving an infant nourishment, but too often the nursing bottle, containing juice, is misused as a pacifier to comfort or control infant behavior.

As soon as an infant has teeth, he is susceptible to tooth decay. The strength and health of his teeth may well depend on bottle-feeding habits that are established as soon as he starts taking juices. If a child is given juice from a bottle, the sugar-rich liquid gathers in pools around his upper teeth; this can eventually cause tooth decay. Nursing-bottle cavities destroy practically all the upper deciduous (baby) teeth because of prolonged contact with juices fed by bottle. The cavities are painful and unattractive, and the teeth may break or become impossible to repair. If primary teeth are lost too early in life, the incoming permanent teeth may be crowded or crooked. The decay or early loss of primary teeth could also cause speech problems later on as well as a poor self-image and loss of appetite (as cold, hot, or hard foods may be difficult or painful to eat). The loss of appetite may eliminate food that is important to a well-balanced diet.

The following points should be kept in mind in preventing nursing-bottle syndrome:

- *Start infants on juice from a cup; never give it from a bottle.*
- *Do not put your child to bed at night with a bottle.* Even milk and formulas containing many nutrients vital to the development of teeth should not be used as a pacifier at nap or bedtime. (Milk does not normally promote decay, but it too can become harmful if allowed to remain in the mouth for long periods.) If your child must have a bottle at naptime, between feedings, at night, or for comfort, give only fresh water.
- Never use a pacifier dipped in honey or other sweeteners.
- Clean the infant's or toddler's teeth properly. Wipe teeth

and gums after each feeding with a damp washcloth or a gauze pad to remove plaque. Continue this practice until all primary teeth have erupted (at about two or two and a half years of age), or until the child is old enough to brush; then use a child's toothbrush with short, rounded bristles (and later also use dental floss).

• A well-balanced diet is important to sustain healthy teeth and gum tissue. Serve a food from each of the four food groups at every meal—milk, protein/meat, vegetable/fruit, bread/cereal.

• Limit foods containing sugar. If you do offer candy, cookies, or other sweets, give them only occasionally at mealtimes, not as snacks. This will limit the number of times the teeth are exposed to the acid that leads to decay.

• Serve a food at the end of each meal that will help clear the mouth of food particles, increase salivary flow, and act as a buffer to neutralize the acid that destroys teeth. Swiss, Monterey Jack, or Cheddar cheeses, as well as raw apples, carrots, and celery, are all good choices.

• Start the habit of visiting the dentist for regular checkups at around the child's second birthday.

• Keep in mind that the use of fluoridated drinking water has been found to help prevent cavities.

The following statement was issued by the American Academy of Pediatrics and the American Academy of Pedodontists:

The use of juices from a bottle should be discouraged; infants should be offered juice from a cup as soon as possible. Nursing bottle caries can be avoided if milk in a bottle is not used as a pacifier at nap or bedtime, if milk bottle feeding is discontinued soon after the first birthday, and if juice is always offered from a cup.

CHILDHOOD OBESITY

According to recent surveys and statistics, obesity in school-age children has increased steadily during the last ten years. Several factors contribute to this serious problem: lack of exercise, inactivity because of excessive television watching, an increase in fast-food consumption, genes, and changing life-styles.

The most significant of all these factors is diet. There appears to be no correlation between a baby's weight in the first twelve months and obesity in later years, and it is important *not* to cut back on his intake of calories and fat by diluting formula, giving low-fat or skim milk, or restricting healthy foods and snacks during the first two years. In fact, to do so could cause inadequate growth and weight gain.

Infants under two require more fat in their diets than older children, but if you are concerned that your child is overweight at two years of age, consult your pediatrician or registered dietitian. This is an especially wise thing to do should there be a history of obesity or heart disease in the family.

If a child has a healthy, balanced, and varied diet, started at age one, with proportionate servings from all four basic food groups, severe food-related problems and disease in later life can be avoided.

As a guideline, the average child can be expected to eat one tablespoonful of food from each food group at each meal for each year of its age.

You will notice that cookies, ice cream, pies, cakes, candy, chocolate, hot dogs, potato chips, and fast foods are not on this table, and should not be part of your child's daily food requirement. They can, however, be offered sparingly on special occasions, so long as the emphasis is on a balanced diet from the four food groups.

The concern should be on making the entire pattern sound. It is important to lay the foundation for a varied and healthy diet. Good eating habits and a nutritious diet will go a long

THE FOUR FOOD GROUPS			
Milk Group 3–4 servings/ day	*Meat Group 2 servings/ day*	*Vegetable/ Fruit Group 4 servings/day*	*Grains 4 servings/ day*
Cheese	Beans/	Apple	Bagel
Milk	Nuts	Apricot	Bread
Yogurt	Beef	Avocado	Cereal
	Chicken	Banana	Crackers
	Eggs	Beets	Muffin
	Fish	Berries	Pasta
	Lamb	Broccoli	Rice
	Pork	Brussels	
	Tofu	sprouts	
	Turkey	Cabbage	
		Carrots	
		Cauliflower	
		Corn	
		Figs	
		Grapefruit	
		Green beans	
		Kiwi	
		Orange	
		Papaya	
		Peach	
		Pear	
		Peas	
		Potatoes	
		Pumpkin	
		Spinach	
		Squash	
		Tomatoes	
		Yams	

way toward reducing the possibility of your child suffering from weight problems later in life.

Here are some preventive measures worth adopting for your baby:

- Don't sweeten cereals. If you don't start using sugar on cereals, your baby will get used to the basic taste and will not demand sweeteners.
- If your baby will not accept cereals, try adding fresh fruit such as bananas, apples, pears, peaches, or prunes. These will also provide important vitamins and minerals.
- Don't insist on your child eating every last spoonful. You don't know the extent of his appetite for that meal, so watch carefully for the first sign that he has had enough.
- Don't get angry or upset when your baby's attention is distracted, when food is spat out, rubbed in the hair or high chair, and his mouth clamps shut. You are being told, "Enough, thank you," and it is important for you to listen to the message. Quietly remove all food, or mealtimes may become a battleground for attention as well as a test of wills, which is the last thing you want.
- If your child is hurt or unhappy, don't comfort him with food or candy. Give him love, hugs, and kisses. One of the hardest habits to avoid is giving your baby a bottle to quiet him down. But if you don't start the habit, you won't have to break it.
- Don't be fanatical about never allowing your little one to have cakes, cookies, or candies. A good rule is to allow sweets on special occasions such as holidays and birthdays. They should not be allowed on a daily basis. If your infant has not been totally deprived of sweets, he is not likely to rebel and go to the other extreme as an adult. (An added bonus to this rule is that treats given only occasionally seem to give even greater pleasure as something very special.)
- Turkey and chicken are most recommended for babies. Serve beef, lamb, pork, and ham less frequently. Choose lean cuts of meat. Trim all visible fat before cooking. Use the following meats very sparingly: organ meats, mutton,

spareribs, frankfurters, sausages, fatty hamburgers, bacon, luncheon meat, and heavily marbled meats.
- Bake, broil, microwave, or steam food rather than fry it.
- Avoid frequent use of gravies and sauces made with butter, fats, or cream. Don't use commercial coating mixes, as they contain large amounts of sugar and fat.
- Children love pasta and bread, good carbohydrates that should be encouraged, together with other grains, fruits, vegetables, and legumes.

ALLERGIES

Food allergies are very common among infants, toddlers, and children, but are sometimes very difficult to diagnose. A doctor should always be consulted to correctly identify any allergy, as a wrong diagnosis could eliminate important staple foods from the diet, thereby preventing the child from receiving optimal nutrition.

Before starting a baby on solids, the parents should check both sides of the family to ascertain if there are tendencies toward allergies to specific foods. If so, those foods should be avoided until after the child is one year of age.

Many infants show intolerance toward certain foods either because their digestive systems are insufficiently developed or because of allergic reactions. When introducing a new food into an infant's diet, watch carefully for any negative reaction, such as diarrhea, vomiting, fever, rash, swelling, or itching. Always wait at least four days before introducing another new food so that the problem food can be easily identified if a reaction should occur.

The following list shows foods commonly known to cause

allergies or intolerance in babies, and the suggested time to introduce them into the diet. If any reaction is noted, discontinue feeding *immediately* and consult a doctor.

Possible Allergy/Intolerance Food	May be offered at . . .
Milk, milk products (i.e., cheese, yogurt, etc.), egg yolk	Six months
Wheat, buckwheat, semolina, citrus fruits and juices, cooked tomatoes	Eight months
Fish, shellfish, egg whites, peanuts and other nuts,* corn, berries, raw tomatoes, cocoa, chocolate	Latter part of the first year

*Note: As nuts are potential choke foods, they should be introduced to the infant in the form of nut butters.

INTRODUCING SOLIDS

Fifty years ago the most common age to introduce solid foods to babies was twelve months. Twenty-five years ago pediatricians suggested starting solids and juices at six weeks. Today, the consensus is that six months is the right time. At this age, most of an infant's supply of iron has been used up and, since neither human nor cow's milk contains an adequate amount of iron, an infant who is fed only milk may develop anemia.

Until a baby is six months of age, the enzymes in his system are equipped to digest only mother's milk or a reasonably close substitute. At six months, however, the necessary enzymes are developed so that a baby can digest solid food.

Solids given too early may lessen a baby's appetite for milk or formula and rob him of essential nutrients. According to the American Academy of Pediatrics, children who are fed semisolids prior to four to six months of age are not advanced nutritionally or developmentally and, in fact, may be hindered because of their reduced intake of milk. Many doctors and nutritionists also feel that food introduced earlier than six months may cause allergic reactions in sensitive children.

There are differences of opinion about whether to feed solids before nursing or bottle feeding or afterward. One theory suggests introducing solid food when your baby is hungry and will be more eager to accept it; another is that if the baby is really hungry and waiting for the breast or bottle, but is offered a spoon with strange-tasting stuff on it, he will be furious and want no part of it. Choose the method you feel is best. Tune in to your little one and listen, feel, and observe all he is telling you, even though he cannot talk. Remember, you know your baby better than anyone else.

Be patient and understanding. Until now, sucking has been all your child has needed to satisfy his hunger. Suddenly he has to figure out how to get this unusually flavored and textured mixture off a spoon and into his mouth. No easy task, and some of the food will cover a much wider territory than his mouth for a while. If you can look at these first attempts at feeding as fun and not be nervous, it will be an adventure. You will both improve with practice.

Use a slim, shallow spoon and always try to put the spoon *on* your baby's tongue. Start with small servings (about ½ tablespoonful) and take your time. However, don't spend more than twenty to thirty minutes on each meal. Relax and enjoy, as the mood you establish at this point is as important as the food you are teaching your child to eat.

If some foods need thinning down, and your infant cannot or will not tolerate pasteurized cow's milk, use your breast milk. Alternatively, you can give him goat milk or soy milk products, which are easily digested, or use formula or juice. Keep all cooked food temperatures between tepid and warm. Test each dish yourself first, as hot food is frightening and may burn your baby's mouth.

What should baby's first meal consist of?

Talk to your pediatrician first and follow his suggestions. However, there are several good choices to consider, including rice cereal (which is easy to digest), very ripe, finely mashed banana or pear, and applesauce. Some doctors recommend introducing cooked, puréed strained vegetables before fruits, as they are blander. If you decide to do this, start with "yellow" vegetables, such as carrots, potatoes, squash, and sweet potatoes. (In the next couple of months you may add beets, peas, spinach, green beans, asparagus, cauliflower, and avocados.)

Should your baby refuse to take a food you are giving him for the first time, don't agonize over it or insist. Try something else. Once he is more used to coping with solids, he will probably be much more amenable toward previously rejected foods.

If you started with rice cereal, for instance, and your child has tolerated it well for several days, introduce him to oatmeal. Don't use the adult variety but one prepared especially for infants. If he tolerates oatmeal well, follow it with barley cereal.

When introducing any new food, give it to your child for at least four days. Once you see that he is tolerating it well, and that he has no allergic reaction to it, you may introduce something else. In the event of intolerance or allergy to a specific food, you may find one or more of the following symptoms: change in amount and smell of food baby spits up, frequent and runny stools, rashes, fever, or vomiting. Call your doctor immediately should any of these symptoms occur and work out a special diet with him.

Feed solids only once a day initially; in the morning is best. After a week of cereal for breakfast, add an evening feeding, too. Cereal should now be fed to your little one daily until he is at least eighteen months old. Remember, though, nursing or the bottle is still going to be his main source of food, and it will be at least another month before he is eating a complete meal.

About four weeks after introducing cereals, fruit, and vegetables, meat may be added to the diet. As your baby drinks less milk, meat will provide most of his protein, iron, and the

B complex vitamins. All meats should be finely ground or strained so they can be easily swallowed. Use chicken, turkey, lamb, and beef. Pork, although very high in protein, is also very high in fat and should not be given too often. When it is served, it must be very well cooked.

Here are some other guidelines to keep in mind while weaning your baby:

- Don't feed excessive amounts of juice. This may decrease your baby's intake of milk or formula, which is still his most important nutrient.
- Don't add sugar or honey to any cereal. If your baby doesn't get used to sweet tastes, he won't miss them.
- When you decide to introduce fruits or vegetables into the diet, use the same procedure as for cereal—only one fruit or vegetable at a time. Bananas must be very ripe—the skin should be speckled brown—as unripe bananas are difficult to digest. Other fruits you may give your baby at this time are cooked apples, pears, prunes, peaches, and apricots.
- Most fruits, and especially prunes, have a mild laxative effect, so keep this in mind if your baby is constipated. You can increase or decrease the amount of fruit you give, depending on the frequency and consistency of your baby's bowel movements. Of course, there will be a change in baby's bowel movements once you start feeding him solids. This is normal. A breast-fed baby will probably have more frequent movements once he is started on solids, although this is not necessarily true of a bottle-fed baby.
- Don't put your child to bed with a bottle of juice or milk once his teeth start coming through. This may quite possibly promote cavities. If he needs the comfort of sucking occasionally after you have put him to bed, give him a bottle of plain boiled water.

SUMMARY: WHEN TO
INTRODUCE SOLIDS

Six Months

Juices   Apple, apricot nectar, carrot (in moderation),
                    pear, and prune
Fruits   Cooked apples, apricots, nectarines,
                    peaches, pears, plums, and prunes; raw,
                    very ripe bananas, nectarines, and peaches
Vegetables   Carrots, green beans, fresh peas, potatoes,
                    sweet potatoes, wax beans, winter squash,
                    and yams (all cooked)
Miscellaneous   Cereals, except wheat

Seven Months

Juices   Cherry
Fruits   Cooked pitted cherries; raw, very ripe
                    papaya and pears
Vegetables   Broccoli, celery, summer squash, and
                    zucchini (all cooked)
Miscellaneous   Tofu

Eight Months

Fruits   Ripe apricots, plums, and prunes (all raw)
Vegetables   Asparagus, beets, corn, greens, legumes
                    (beans, peas, lentils), okra, parsnips,
                    peppers, rutabaga, spinach, tomatoes, and
                    turnips (all cooked)
Miscellaneous   Cheese, egg yolk, meats, and yogurt

Nine to Eleven Months

Juices · · · · · · · · · Cranberry, grape, grapefruit, guava nectar, lemon, mango nectar, orange, papaya nectar, pineapple, and tomato

Although citrus fruits (oranges, grapefruits, lemons, limes) can be allergenic, they are an excellent source of vitamin C. Therefore, citrus juices may be introduced at this time. Dilute them with an equal amount of water until you are satisfied that your baby shows no sign of allergic reaction.

Fruits · · · · · · · · · Avocado, cantaloupe, pitted cherries, guava, kiwi fruit, mangoes, persimmons, and pineapple (all raw)

Vegetables · · · · · · Brussels sprouts, cabbage, cauliflower, eggplant, and kohlrabi (all cooked)

Miscellaneous · · · Tuna; wheat products

Twelve Months

Fruits · · · · · · · · · Berries, figs, grapes, grapefruit, and oranges (all raw)

Vegetables · · · · · · Mushrooms and onions; raw cucumber (peeled), and raw tomatoes

Miscellaneous · · · Egg white; fish

NOTES · · · · · · · · · (1) Never boil juices. Heat destroys vitamin C.
(2) Except where specified raw, all vegetables should be cooked during the first year.

HOMEMADE BABY FOODS

Why make your own baby foods when they can be purchased from the market? There are many advantages, some of which are:

- They are freshly made and more nutritious.
- They cost less than commercial baby foods.
- They can be made to different consistencies, to suit your baby's needs. Many commercial baby foods are too thin for older infants.
- They can be familiar foods, prepared without excess water or salt, sugar, starches, or tapioca (which are often added to store-bought baby foods).
- Baby is introduced to foods that taste more like the table foods he will soon be eating.
- Homemade baby food need take no longer to prepare than heating a jar of the commercial kind. Many baby foods can be prepared in a few minutes or even less using the microwave oven.

Here are some points to remember when preparing baby foods at home:

- Clean hands, utensils, and work surfaces are essential. Wash all equipment thoroughly in hot soapy water and rinse well before using. Take apart food grinders, blenders, and processors after each use and wash them thoroughly. Dry each part before putting appliance together again.
- Use fresh, good-quality food that has been stored in clean containers at correct refrigerator temperatures (no higher than 40°F [4°C]). Vegetables (especially spinach) should be fresh and used within two days of purchase.
- Wash all fruits, vegetables, fish, meats (except for red or ground meats), and poultry before preparing.
- Do not overcook vegetables or fruits. Either cook them in a small amount of water in a covered pan or, whenever possible microwave or steam them, saving the liquid for thinning the food. Cook just until tender.
- Put leftovers in clean covered containers and refrigerate immediately. Use within one or two days.
- To freeze baby food, pour portions into individual plastic ice cube trays. When frozen, pop food cubes out of containers into a plastic bag, seal, and store in freezer. To serve, remove a cube and melt over low heat in a small saucepan, or

defrost in a microwave. Freezer temperature should be 0°F (−18°C) or lower. Use frozen baby foods within two months.

- Heat only the quantity of food you need for each feeding whenever possible. Leftovers from the feeding dish should be discarded.
- When preparing family recipes for baby, remove his portion before adding salt, sugar, or spicy seasonings.

EQUIPMENT (SEE ALSO "BASIC EQUIPMENT LIST," WHICH FOLLOWS)

Infant foods can be prepared with many kinds of equipment, from a simple fork, sieve, or strainer to an expensive food processor. Food mills, baby-food grinders, and blenders may also be used, and they work well. If using a wire strainer, be sure it is in very good condition so that there is no danger of small pieces of mesh getting into the food.

PREPARING CEREALS

Most infants start out with precooked baby cereals, fortified with iron. Those are simply prepared by stirring dry cereal into the appropriate quantity of warmed liquid.

Health-food stores now carry a wide variety of unrefined, quick-cooking cereals such as oat, cream of rye, cream of soya, cream of wheat, cream of rice, and corn grits, none of which take more than a few minutes to cook. Also available are whole-grain cereals, which usually require approximately thirty minutes to cook (and may need to be puréed before being served to infants). These cereals include rolled oats, millet, barley flakes, rice, and cracked wheat. Cooking directions can be found on the packages. But remember that these cereals contain much less iron than commercial infant cereals, and that breast milk and cow's milk contain very little iron. From the age of six months, an infant may require additional iron in his diet, and this should be checked with a pediatrician.

PREPARING VEGETABLES

Wash and peel vegetables, cut into small even-sized pieces, and microwave, steam, or boil in a small amount of water until soft. (Carrots should be scrubbed, not peeled, to retain nutrients.)

Most vegetables cook in a few minutes and then can be pressed through a fine strainer, mashed with a fork, or puréed. Remove any coarse pieces or skin. If using a blender or food processor, mix ½ cup of cooked, diced vegetables with ¼ cup of liquid (milk, vegetable or meat broth, formula, or juice). Blend until smooth.

PREPARING FRUITS

Prepare and cook fresh fruits as for vegetables, preferably peeling fruits *after* cooking. Bananas should be ripe, never cooked, and need only be mashed with a fork to serve. Stew or microwave dried fruits in a little water until soft, then purée in the cooking liquid for infants, or mash for older children. Pitted dried fruits can be offered as a finger food at twelve months without being soaked or cooked.

PREPARING MEATS AND FISH

Cut lean raw beef, lamb, chicken, turkey, or fish into small pieces, then steam, microwave, bake, broil, stew, or sauté; then purée or grind meat in a food mill or grinder, blender, or processor. After meat or fish is cooked, liquid may be used for thinning.

Once an infant has several teeth, the consistency of foods should be coarser but still tender. Mash fruits and vegetables, finely chop meats, progressing to finely diced meats.

SAVING TIME

Preparing baby foods may seem too time-consuming for working parents. But keeping in mind the child's well-being, compromises can be worked out to make it possible to prepare nutritious homemade baby foods quickly and easily for later use. Home-cooked vegetables, fruits, and eggs can be made very quickly and served with commercial baby meat dishes that would take a little longer to prepare yourself.

To take on outings or for baby-sitters, small lunch-box thermos bottles are ideal for storing soft steamed or microwaved vegetables and fruits. The food can be mashed either prior to being put in the thermos or just before serving.

Several kinds of vegetables can be microwaved or steamed together, some to serve now, some for later. When an infant can cope with more textured foods, use several small thermos "pots" for pasta, rice, beans, cottage cheese, yogurt, fruit, meats, or vegetables. In this way, it is possible for your baby to be given the nutritious foods you have prepared even if you cannot be there to feed him yourself.

BASIC EQUIPMENT LIST (ONE OR MORE OF THE FOLLOWING):

Small sieve or strainer
Food mill or grinder
Food processor or blender
Potato masher
Steamer basket or saucepan with steamer
Lidded saucepan
Egg poacher (for reheating leftovers)
Small covered containers for leftovers
Individual ice cube trays for freezing food (optional)
Storage bags for freezing (optional)
Measuring spoons, 1-teaspoon and 1-tablespoon sizes
Paring knife
Vegetable brush

Babies' and Toddlers' Balanced Menus

BREAKFASTS

In the first year of your baby's life, breakfasts are rather simple, with the emphasis on cereals. The most suitable cereals are rice, oats, barley, rye, and millet. The specially prepared infant cereals available in supermarkets are best initially, as they are fortified with iron and do not contain sugar or salt. Breast milk, formula, cow's milk, or juice can be used to mix the cereals.

In addition to cereals, serve mashed banana, applesauce, or puréed, cooked fresh pears, peaches, or apricots. These fruits can be mixed with cereal or offered separately. If you don't give your baby fruit, give him instead a cup of apple, pear, apricot, or cherry juice. One egg *yolk*, hard-boiled or scrambled with a tablespoon of milk, will make this a nutritionally complete breakfast.

After twelve months, breakfasts become more diversified. The menus that follow will give you some ideas to supplement with your own.

When I started my daughter on wheat cereals, I found two varieties at the health-food store that were instant favorites. The first was a Swiss cereal containing rye, oat, and millet flakes, whole wheat, dried shredded dates, apples, bananas, ground almonds, and wheat germ. I served it cold with milk. The second was a sprouted-wheat cereal with bananas which also contained oats and barley. Later I switched to regular oatmeal, and I tried other cereals such as grits, Roman Meal, and Malt-O-Meal, which my little one enjoyed. Your baby will choose his own favorites. Introduce him to many kinds but always read the labels first to ensure the cereals do not contain sugar or salt. Stay away from ready-to-eat commercial cereals, as most of them contain enormous amounts of sugar (some more than 50 percent) and large quantities of salt (up to 375 milligrams per ounce). Many of these cereals also contain BHA and BHT, antioxidants that help preserve freshness.

Your baby should have cooked cereal at least once a day until he is eighteen months old. For a special treat you can occasionally replace cereal with pancakes (I found a soy-wheat pancake mix that is naturally sweet, as it contains dried apples and pear juice), or whole wheat toast spread with mashed banana or cheese.

After twelve months is also the time to introduce brewer's yeast into your infant's juice at breakfast. It is a superior source of the natural B complex vitamins. Start with ⅛ teaspoon and slowly increase the quantity to 1 teaspoon.

A few final facts on cereals that are important to keep in mind: All cereals contain some protein, approximately 2 to 6 grams per ounce, but are low in lysine, an essential amino acid. However, the addition of milk, which is rich in lysine, will make the cereal protein complete. Governmental dietary guidelines recommend that Americans reduce their intake of fats and consume more complex carbohydrates such as corn, wheat, rice, oats, and barley, the main ingredients of cereals. According to these guidelines, a bowl of *unsweetened* cereal is healthier than fried eggs and bacon.

12 Months Onward

Note: Soft-boiled eggs should be boiled for at least 5 minutes.
*See Index for recipes.

Soft-boiled egg
Oatmeal with Applesauce*
and milk
½ cup orange juice with 1
tsp. brewer's yeast

———

Millet Cereal* with
Applesauce*
½ cup orange juice with 1
tsp. brewer's yeast

———

Roman Meal cereal with
milk
½ fresh peach, sliced

———

Scrambled egg
½ slice whole wheat bread
and butter with banana
slices
1 cup milk

———

Cornmeal Mush* with milk
½ banana
1 cup warm milk with carob

———

Hominy grits with milk
Small piece of melon

———

Swiss cereal with milk
Yogurt
¼ apple, peeled and cored

———

Small soy-wheat pancake
with butter and Applesauce*
Apricot Breakfast Shake*

———

Rice cereal with milk
Poached egg
½ apple or pear, peeled and
cored

———

Hominy grits with butter
and milk
½ banana
½ cup apple juice with 1 tsp.
brewer's yeast

———

Sprouted cereal with milk
Blueberry Muffin*
Orange slices

———

Barley cereal with milk
Fresh strawberries
½ cup orange juice with
1 tsp. brewer's yeast

———

Malt-O-Meal with milk
Poached egg
¼ pear, peeled and cored

————

Small soy-wheat pancake
with butter and banana
Orange Milk Whip*

————

Oatmeal with fresh
strawberries and milk
String cheese

————

Swiss cereal with milk
Poached egg
½ cup fresh carrot juice

————

Bread Pudding* with raisins
½ cup orange juice with
1 tsp. brewer's yeast

————

Swedish Potato Pancake*
with Applesauce*
1 cup milk

————

Rye cereal with milk
Scrambled egg
Orange Milk Whip*

————

Cornmeal Mush* with milk
Orange slices
Apricot Breakfast Shake*

————

Cottage cheese
½ slice whole wheat toast
with nut butter
½ cup orange juice with
1 tsp. brewer's yeast

LUNCH AND DINNER MENUS

The menus that follow are samples that provide nutritious and balanced meals. Lunches and dinners are interchangeable and may be served either at midday or in the evening. Give your baby ½ tablespoonful of food from each food group at six months of age and progress to 1 tablespoonful at around a year. If your baby's appetite is larger, increase the amounts equally from the four food groups to satisfy it.

All the menus for the first twelve months you can continue to use later. Only the quantity and consistency of the food change, depending on baby's age and the number of teeth he has.

I usually served my child only one meat dish a day, and many days I served no meat at all, making up the protein requirement with egg yolk, cheese, yogurt, milk, and rice and beans. By her first birthday she had shown no signs of allergies, so I fed her the food I prepared for the rest of my family. There was some increase in her salt intake, but it was very moderate. For our welfare as well as my daughter's, I have cut down drastically on salt in our diets.

Many of the meals listed here can be prepared very quickly. Others, such as those comprising soups, casseroles, beans, and roasts, can be made in a crockpot, with leftovers used on working days. And of course as time went on, Mirabai had her small share of what I cooked for the rest of the family.

Vegetables are always more nutritious and attractive if freshly steamed or microwaved, as needed. Steaming or microwaving takes only a few minutes.

Menu dishes requiring a special recipe are marked with an asterisk (*). See the Index for page numbers. As noted in the menus, all meals should be accompanied by nursing, formula, or milk.

A steamer and a blender or food processor are fine investments if you don't already have them. If you don't have a microwave, I strongly recommend using the steamer for your own as well as your baby's foods. An egg poacher is also useful for reheating small portions of up to three or four different foods quickly and easily.

When cooking fruit, I prepared and puréed enough for three or four days, then refrigerated it in sterilized baby jars. Bottles can be sterilized in a dishwasher, or by boiling them in a saucepan of water for five minutes.

I did not freeze my baby foods because it usually took as long to heat them as it did to prepare them from scratch. I also felt that some of the flavor was lost by freezing. This, however, is an individual preference and freezing should not be discounted if you find it useful.

Seven Months

*Note: Each meal should be accompanied
by nursing, formula, or milk.
See Index for recipes.

Creamed summer squash
Mashed peas
Mashed pear

————

Puréed broccoli
Rice and Prune Pudding*

————

Creamed string beans
Sweet Potato and Apple
Purée*

————

Creamed carrots and
zucchini
Mashed banana

————

Mashed potato
Mashed peas
Applesauce*

————

Creamed squash
Mashed green beans
Mashed peeled nectarine

————

Mashed carrots and peas
Cooked Barley,* mashed
Mashed pear

————

Puréed wax beans
Mashed banana

————

Mashed broccoli
Rice
Mashed plum and tofu

————

Mashed potato and peas
Cooked puréed apricot

————

Mashed tofu
Mashed carrots and green
beans
Mashed pear

————

Mashed sweet potato
Fruit Compote*

————

Mashed sautéed tofu
Creamed green beans
Mashed banana

————

Baked Acorn or Summer
Squash*
Puréed cherries with tofu

———

Puréed carrots
Rice
Mashed peach

———

Mashed carrots and peas
Pastina
Mashed papaya

———

Mashed sweet potato
Mashed pitted plum and
banana with tofu

———

Mashed potatoes and peas
Rice and Apricot Pudding*

———

Creamed carrots
Boiled potato, mashed with
butter
Applesauce*

———

Creamed broccoli
Carrot Apple Purée*

———

Baked Acorn Squash*
Plum Yum*

Eight Months

*Note: Each meal should be accompanied
by nursing, formula, or milk.
See Index for recipes.

Creamed spinach
Mashed yam
ABC Dessert*

———

Leftover Turkey Soup* with
vegetables
Peachy Pudding*

———

Small White Beans* (with
tomato and parsley)
Cottage Cheese Pudding*

———

Pastina with Peas*
Ricotta cheese with mashed
peach

———

Vegetables Tofu*
Mashed peas
Plain yogurt with mashed
pear

———

Yam Soup*
Mashed pinto beans
Rice and Prune Pudding*

———

Puréed beef
Steamed yellow squash,
mashed
Creamed string beans
Applesauce*

———

Lentil and Banana Mash*
Rice Royal*
Plain yogurt

———

Mashed broccoli and carrots
Rice
Ricotta cheese with mashed
peach

———

Sweet Potato and Apple
Purée*
Mashed Spinach

———

Frijoles II* (refried beans)
Apple Mist*

———

Mashed Cuban Black Beans*
(and rice)
Carrot Apple Purée*
Plain yogurt

———

Lentil Roast*
Rice Pudding*

———

Puréed chicken
Mashed Rutabaga and
Carrots*
Mashed banana

———

Stelline with Cottage
Cheese*
Cream of Tomato Soup*
Fruit Compote*

———

Vegetable Custard*
Mashed apricots and tofu

———

Beans and Broccoli with
Stars*
Carrots and Beets with
Apple*

———

Tofu-Rice Casserole*
Baked Acorn Squash*
Grape Divine*

———

Macaroni Marinara*
Tofu with Egg*
Carrot Apple Purée*

———

Puréed turkey
Baked sweet potato, mashed
Mashed pear

———

Lentil and Potato Stew*
Broiled Tomato*
Rice Pudding*

———

Shepherd's Pie*
Mashed peas
Mashed banana

———

Puréed split peas
Heavenly Potato*
Mashed Rutabaga and
Carrots*
Plum Yum*

———

Vegetable Custard*
Cooked Rice*
Stewed Plums* (with
yogurt)

Nine Months

*Note: Each meal should be accompanied
by nursing, formula, or milk.
See Index for recipes.

Microwave Baked Potato
Sautéed ground beef
Papaya slices

———

Spinach Yogurt Bake*
Baked sweet potato
Peeled pear slices

———

Cheesy Baked Squash*
Mashed black-eyed peas
Peeled, pitted peach slices

———

Finely shredded turkey
Rice
Green Peas with Pineapple*

———

Carrots and Beets with
Apple*
Plain yogurt

———

Stelline with Marinara
Sauce*
Ricotta cheese with apricot

———

Chicken Fricassee*
Cauliflower and carrots,
chopped
Boiled potato
Pineapple pieces

———

Stuffed Tomato Treat*
Rice
Tropical Treat*

———

Cooked Barley* (with
ground beef)
Chopped carrots with
parsley
Melon slices

———

Broiled ground beef
Baked sweet potato
Steamed broccoli
Peeled pitted nectarine slices

———

Finely chopped turkey
Steamed chopped carrots
Rice and Pineapple
Pudding*

———

Norwegian Lamb and
Cabbage*
Boiled potato
Cantaloupe slices

———

Tofu-Rice Casserole*
Tomato Eggplant Cups*
Banana Raita*

———

Homemade Chicken Soup*
(with pastina and carrots)
Bread Pudding*

———

Beef, Bean, and Macaroni
Casserole*
Brussels Sprouts and
Carrots in Lemon Butter*
Mango slices

———

Shredded chicken
Yam and Carrot Balls with
Raisins*

———

Cheese and Lentil Loaf*
Avocado and Papaya Salad*

———

Bean and Cheese Melt*
Steamed chopped spinach
Yogurt Ambrosia*

———

Broiled ground lamb
Heart of artichoke
Rice
Orange Cloud*

———

Mashed potato
Creamy Turnip*
Mango slices

———

Stuffed Bell Peppers*
Peruvian Bean Purée*
Bread Pudding*

Tofu and Cauliflower*
Avocado and tomato slices
Banana Coconut Pudding*

Sweet Potato and Apple
Purée*
Mashed peas

Zucchini Beef Skillet*
Carrots and Beets with
Apple*

Eggplant Parmesan*
Rice
Plain yogurt with papaya
slices

Frijoles I* (refried beans)
Yam and Carrot Balls with
Raisins*
Rice Royal*
Plain yogurt with peach
slices

Baked Acorn Squash*
Rice Pudding*

Ten Months

*Note: Each meal should be accompanied
by nursing, formula, or milk.
See Index for recipes.

Microwave asparagus
Rice Royal*
ABC Dessert*

Baked Mostaccioli*
Avocado and Papaya Salad*

Split Pea Soup*
Slice whole wheat bread
Rice Pudding*

Roast Lamb and Potatoes*
Green Peas with Pineapple*

Soy Potato Burgers*
Creamy Turnip*
Kiwi fruit slices

Leftover Lamb with Beans*
Mashed Rutabaga and
Carrots*
Sliced fresh pear

Cream of Broccoli Soup*
Slice whole wheat bread
Cottage Cheese Pudding*

———

Scalloped Potatoes with
Ham*
Asparagus with Parmesan
Cheese*
Apple Gel*

———

Vegetables Tofu*
Bean and Cheese Melt*
Broiled Banana*

———

Meatballs*
Heavenly Potato*
Green Peas with Pineapple*

———

Stelline with Cottage
Cheese*
Steamed broccoli
Avocado and tomato slices
Baked apple*

———

Finely diced chicken
Mashed potato
Chopped spinach
Banana Coconut Pudding*

———

Karin's Health Soup*
Slice whole wheat toast
Yogurt Ambrosia*

———

Chicken Soup with Speck*
Slice whole wheat bread
Tropical Treat*

———

Meat Cakes*
Sweet Potato Scramble*
Mashed avocado and
banana

———

Tofu-Cheese Soufflé*
Cooked beets and green
beans
Sliced apple

———

Yam and Carrot Balls with
Raisins*
Cantaloupe slices with
yogurt

———

Syrian Lentil Soup*
Slice whole wheat bread
Stewed Plums* (with plain
yogurt)

———

Microwave Chicken Breast*
Cooked beets and Brussels
sprouts
Rice and Apricot Pudding*

———

Cream of Tomato Soup*
Sweet and Savory Eggplant*
Rice
Peach slices

Yam Soup*
Corn Bread*
Avocado and Papaya Salad*
Banana Raita*

Small White Beans*
Mashed carrots
Grape Divine*

Tomato Eggplant Cups*
Cottage cheese with mango
slices

Cold Cream of Avocado
Soup*
Vegetable Rice Casserole*
Poached Apple*

Eleven Months

*Note: Each meal should be accompanied
by nursing, formula, or milk.
See Index for recipes.

Tofu and Cauliflower*
Green Peas with Pineapple*
Apple Gel*

Meatballs*
Mashed potato
Chopped carrots and green
beans
Pear Surprise*

Yellow Pea Soup with
Vegetables and Sausage*
Banana

Stelline with Cottage
Cheese*
Steamed carrots and peas
Yogurt Ambrosia*

Baked Chicken with
Tarragon*
Creamed corn
Rice
Watermelon

Chicken Soup with Speck*
Avocado and tomato slices
Papaya with cottage cheese

Millet Soufflé*
Stuffed Tomato Treat*
Cold Apricot Soup*

———

Turkey sausage, chopped
Swedish Potato Pancakes*
with Applesauce*
Mashed Rutabaga and
Carrots*

———

Cheese and Lentil Loaf*
Squash with Green Beans*
Cottage cheese with peach
slices

———

Beans, Rice, and Vegetable
Soup*
Peachy Pudding*

———

Lentil Soup*
Rice Royal*
Summer Delight*

———

Piselli con Uova* (peas
with egg)
Rice
Slice whole wheat bread
Banana Raita*

———

Lima Beans*
Rice
Sweet Potato Scramble*
Persimmon slices

———

Megan's Favorite Chicken
Soup*
Apple slices
Slice whole wheat bread

———

Couscous with Mixed
Vegetables*
Nectarine slices
Yogurt

———

Vegetable Tofu*
Rice
Brussels Sprouts and
Carrots in Lemon Butter*
Kiwi Kwiki*

———

Groundnut Chicken Stew*
Rice
Broiled Banana*

———

Sweet Potato Scramble*
Rice and Apricot Pudding*

———

Tofu-Rice Casserole*
Broiled Tomato*
Apple Mist*

———

Pasta e Fagioli* (macaroni
and beans)
Steamed spinach
Cantaloupe slices

Asparagus Omelet*
Steamed zucchini and
carrots
Sautéed potato
Cold Melon Soup*

———

Rice with Cheese*
Carrots and Beets with
Apple*
ABC Dessert*

———

Cottage Cheese and Noodle
Casserole*
Avocado and tomato slices
Slice whole wheat bread
Applesauce* (with plain
yogurt)

Twelve Months

Note: Each meal should be accompanied by milk.
*See Index for recipes.

Small sticks of cold ham
Garbanzo Bean Purée*
Pita Bread*
Cold, cooked carrot sticks
Figs in Yogurt*

———

Cabbage Rolls*
Green Beans with Walnuts*
Apricot Soup*

———

Oven-Baked Fish*
Baked potato
Mashed steamed carrots
Fresh pear slices

———

Broiled Sturgeon*
Boiled potato
Steamed, chopped spinach
Strawberries

———

Meat Cakes*
Bulgur Pilaf*
Cauliflower with Avocado-
Tahini Dressing*
Tangerine segments

———

Steamed Salmon Loaf*
Mashed potato
Steamed chopped broccoli
Fresh raspberries

———

Pineapple Chicken
Supreme*
Rice
Plain yogurt

———

Fiske Kaker* (Norwegian
fish cakes)
Boiled potato
Cooked beets
Pear Delight*

———

Semolina Primavera*
Ricotta cheese with
strawberries

———

Spinach and Potato
Casserole*
Slice whole wheat bread
Yogurt Delight*

———

Simple Fish and Vegetables*
Rice
Cantaloupe slices

———

Ham Omelet*
Asparagus with Parmesan
Cheese*
Tropical Treat*

———

Fricassee of Chicken*
Carrot Raita*
Fresh pineapple pieces

———

Fried Tofu with
Mushrooms*
Heavenly Potato*
Fresh peach slices

———

Cholent* (meat, bean, and
vegetable soup)
Challah* (bread)
Sliced seeded orange

———

Egg Scramble*
Baked sweet potato
Peas
Fruit Compote*

———

Chicken and Papaya Soup*
Slice whole wheat bread
Kiwi fruit slices

———

Fish with Fresh Tomato*
Mashed potato
Avocado slices
Strawberry Banana Mold*

———

Macaroni Marinara*
Steamed broccoli and carrots
Rice Pudding*

———

Stuffed Bell Peppers*
Avocado and Papaya Salad*
Cottage Cheese Pudding*

———

Sole Meunière*
Baked potato
Creamy Turnip*
Watermelon pieces

———

Arabian Stew*
Pita Bread*
Persian melon slices

———

Lentil Roast*
Stuffed Tomato Treat*
Cranberry Cubes*

———

Poached Fish with Yogurt
Sauce*
Mashed potato
Green beans
Fresh Fruit Salad*

———

Celery Soup*
Slice whole wheat bread
Tuna fish salad
Orange segments

———

Thirteen to Seventeen Months

Note: Each meal should be accompanied by milk.
*See Index for recipes.

Beef, Bean, and Macaroni
Casserole*
Okra
Persimmon with Grapes*

———

Egg Nest*
Slice whole wheat bread
Strawberry Fruit Soup*

———

Baked Haddock and
Potatoes*
Steamed broccoli
Tomato and cucumber salad
Homemade Apple Pie*

———

Shrimp and Okra Stew*
Rice
Raspberry Tarte*

———

Ricotta Cheese Pancakes*
Pineapple Coleslaw*
Plain yogurt

———

Tuna Fish Casserole*
Steamed green beans
Fruit Compote*

———

Greek Lamb Stew*
Cucumber Salad*
Orange segments

———

Haddock with Egg Butter*
Boiled potato
Steamed carrots
Peach slices

————

Summer Salad*
Pita Bread* (with melted
cheese)

————

Stelline with Cottage
Cheese*
Avocado and Papaya Salad*
Strawberries

————

Scalloped Potatoes with
Ham*
Baked Acorn Squash*
Nectarine slices

————

Poached Egg with Spinach*
Rice Royal*
Apple Strawberry parfait*

————

Fish and Rice Casserole*
Bread Pudding*

————

Black-eyed Peas and Rice*
Yam and Carrot Balls with
Raisins*
Fresh Fruit Salad*

————

Chicken Breasts with Lime
Butter*
Asparagus with Parmesan
Cheese*
Plain yogurt with papaya
slices

————

Crockpot Seafood Chowder*
Carrot Raita*
Poached Apple*

————

Seafood Salad*
Melon Berry Melba*

————

Lentils Indian Style*
Chapatis*
Indian Vegetables with Rice*
Banana Raita*

————

Baked Potatoes with Salmon
Sauce*
Carrot Raita*
Cranberry Cubes*

————

Zucchini Beef Skillet*
Macaroni Marinara*
Pear Surprise*

————

White Bean and Cabbage
Soup*
Slice whole wheat bread
Rice Pudding*

_____

Calamari*
Rice
Tangerine segments

_____

Vegetable Barley Soup*
Slice whole wheat bread
Ricotta cheese and fresh or
canned pineapple pieces

_____

Eighteen Months to Two Years

Note: Each meal should be accompanied by milk.
*See Index for recipes.

Black Bean Soup*
Tabbouleh Salad*
Avocado and Papaya Salad*
Plain yogurt

_____

Quesadilla* (tortilla with
cheese)
Cold Cream of Avocado
Soup*
Rice and Apricot Pudding*

_____

Stir-Fried Squid with
Snow Peas*
Rice
Persimmon

_____

Baked Sea Bass Oriental*
Rice
Stir-fried Chinese pea pods
and mushrooms
Orange segments

_____

Baked Ham in Vegetable
Juice*
Baked yam
Green Beans with Walnuts*
Fresh pineapple pieces

_____

Roast Chicken in Tomato
Sauce*
Mashed potato
Peas
Nectarine slices

_____

Macaroni Salad*
Slice whole wheat bread
Baked Apple*

_____

Cheese Enchiladas*
Frijoles I* (refried beans)
Rice
Kiwi fruit slices

————

Shrimp with Almond Yogurt
Sauce*
Steamed spinach
Rice
Fresh fig

————

Boned Chicken Chinese
Style* (with bean sprouts,
mushrooms, and
snow peas)
Rice
Banana Coconut Pudding*

————

Creamy Halibut Bake*
Baked potato
Steamed asparagus tips
Fresh strawberries

————

Microwave Shepherd's Pie*
Steamed broccoli
Pear slices

————

Italian Rice and Avocado
Salad*
Summer Delight*

————

Tuna Melt*
Steamed asparagus tips
Apple slices

————

Microwave Poached
Chicken Breast*
Sautéed potato
Cantaloupe slices

————

Halloween Stew*
Persimmon and Black
Grapes*

————

Avocado with cooked
shrimp
Half hard-boiled egg and
tomato slices on lettuce leaf
Slice whole wheat bread
Apricot Soup*

————

Cuban Chicken* (with
carrots and potatoes)
Fresh Fruit Salad*

————

Crockpot Chicken with
Tarragon*
Mashed Rutabaga and
Carrots*
Baked potato
ABC Dessert*

————

Asparagus Omelet*
Lentil Soup*
Fresh pitted plum

————

Microwave Mild Curried
Fish
Green beans with yogurt
Fresh pitted cherries

Cream of Tomato Soup*
(with macaroni)
Slice whole wheat bread
Lentil and Banana Mash*
Figs in Yogurt*

Pot-au-Feu*
Norwegian Birthday Cake*

SNACKS AND FINGER FOODS

From about eight months of age, your baby will probably be able to use his thumb and fingers to pick up pieces of food. Although he may have only a couple of teeth, this is a good time to introduce finger foods. These will be "gummed," a little will end up in the tummy, and the remainder will be spat out. Chewing is the first step in your baby's development toward independent feeding.

Start him off with a piece of banana, a rice or rye cracker, thin strips of cheese or avocado, or well-cooked pieces of carrot, potato, apple, or asparagus tips. As your little one acquires more teeth, the list of foods will get longer. After nine months, add wheat bread, wheat crackers, melon, soft raw pitted apricots and prunes. When baby is one year, the fruits you have been cooking, such as apples, pears, and peaches, can be given to him fresh. They must be peeled, cored, and stoned where necessary, and cut into several pieces. Fingers of bread can be covered with cream cheese, apple or banana, thinly sliced cheese, nut butters, mashed carrots, or applesauce.

Make your child's snacks healthy, with food values similar to those of a regular meal. As my daughter ate well at each meal, I usually didn't offer her snacks, although I would give her a cup of milk or juice between meals. If I didn't have time to prepare a hot meal, or she indicated that she was hungry between meals, I made a snack that combined the necessary protein, fats, carbohydrates, vitamins, and minerals. This meant including something from each one of the four food groups listed below:

- *Meat Group:* fish, poultry, eggs, legumes (dried beans, peas, and lentils), nut butters, and tofu
- *Milk Group:* milk, yogurt, and cheeses
- *Fruits and Vegetables Group:* citrus fruits, fleshy fruits, leafy vegetables, green and yellow vegetables, and tubers (potatoes, yams, and other root vegetables)
- *Bread and Cereals Group:* pasta, rice, cereals, cornmeal, oats, grits, and baked goods

Following is a list of snacks that can be easily and quickly prepared from foods that are probably in your refrigerator. I have separated them into three age groups for easy reference.

8 to 12 Months of Age

Hard-boiled egg yolk, ground beef, chicken, turkey, or lamb made into little meat cakes (see page 217)

Mozzarella, jack, Cheddar, Swiss, or string cheese cut into 1 × 3-inch strips; cream cheese on a cracker; yogurt; cottage cheese

Apple, pear, or peach slices, all peeled, cored, and steamed or microwaved until soft; prunes and dried apricots, soaked until soft; ripe bananas

Broccoli, asparagus tips, beets, carrots, cauliflower, peas, string beans, potatoes, turnips, sweet potatoes, cut into 1 × 3-inch pieces (except peas, of course!) and steamed or microwaved; ripe avocado slices

Rye, oat, and rice cereals; toast or crackers. Bread can be hard-
ened for teething by cutting into finger-size pieces and baking in preheated 150° to 200° oven for 15 to 20 minutes.

12 Months to 18 Months

Add to the above:

Whole egg; nut butters; fish sticks; diced or sliced poultry

Fresh fruits, including melon, oranges, figs, mangoes, papaya, kiwi fruit, strawberries, and all other fruits that were
previously cooked

Fresh vegetables, including lettuce, mushroom slices, cut-up
tomatoes, raw broccoli and cauliflower pieces, shredded
carrots, and raw string beans

Whole wheat toast, bread, crackers, and breadsticks. (Make
open-face sandwiches with applesauce, mashed fruits,
melted cheese, or cream cheese.)

18 Months Onward

Milk and fruit shakes, fruit popsicles. *Sample menus:*

Apple wedges with peanut butter. Buttermilk.

Slice of whole wheat bread with cheese. Shredded carrot.
Juice.

Cooked egg with slice of whole wheat bread and butter.
Juice.

Whole wheat crackers. Buttermilk with grated apple.

Open-face banana sandwich on whole wheat bread. Milk.

Mirabai's Diary from Six Months to Her Second Birthday

Mid-September (6 Months)

MIRABAI is six months old today and we are going to celebrate by starting her on solids. I purchased some precooked infant rice cereal, a little of which I mixed with warm milk until it became a semiliquid. I tested the cereal carefully with my lips to make sure it was not too hot. Mirabai was enveloped in a bib stating that "I Love Daddy" and adorned with hearts, pandas, and bluebirds. To complete our exciting initiation into solids, I used a little silver dish that came from Norway a long time ago. However, I bought a modern baby spoon with a white plastic coating over the bowl part.

I cradled Mirabai in my left arm comfortably in a half-sitting position and placed a spoonful of the cereal a little way back on her tongue. She sucked and smacked her lips, the cereal disappeared, and her mouth opened, waiting for the next spoonful. We repeated this procedure until the whole 1½ tablespoonsful were gone. Obviously cereal made a pleasant change for my little one.

The best time to introduce solid or semisolid foods is usually somewhere between five and six months, when several important growth factors exist: breast milk or formula alone is inadequate to support baby's normal growth; iron, which has been stored in the body, becomes depleted; the enzyme necessary to digest foods is present, and the infant's swallowing and chewing reflexes are sufficiently developed.

Learning to eat from a spoon is a very important experience. It may seem temporarily easier to feed semisolids from a bottle with a large-hole nipple, but you will only be delaying your baby's development in feeding. Use a slim baby spoon with no sharp edges. Place a spoonful of food toward the back of the tongue, close to the roof of the mouth, and let the baby do the rest. Rice cereal is good to start with as it is easily digested.

Mirabai has been getting rice cereal for four days now, so today we are going to try barley. I am still using prepared baby cereal, fortified with iron. I have increased the amount to 2 tablespoonsful because her appetite is so good, and there were no ill effects (such as diarrhea, gas, or rashes) from the rice cereal. And she is becoming more adept at getting it off the spoon now.

An aunt in Norway has sent Mirabai a little silver cup, and we are going to try a little apple juice from the cup for the first time. When I offer her the cup, she bites on the rim, and when I tilt it a little, she seems surprised at the cool sweet liquid coming from it. She lowers her head toward the cup again, wanting more.

Rice cereal is the easiest of all cereals for babies to digest, but it is also the lowest in protein. Introducing other varieties, such as oat and barley, is good nutritionally, as well as for getting baby used to different flavors. However, I don't recommend buying the cereals that are premixed with fruit (such as banana). These products have too . much sugar and other sweeteners in them, and it would be better to use fresh mashed banana or other cooked mashed fruits.

Many dentists feel that as soon as an infant's teeth start coming through, juices should be given only from a cup, as this helps prevent cavities that could develop if a bottle is used. (Fruit juices lose their vitamin content if they are heated and should be given at room temperature.) There are several kinds of baby cups. Some have lids with drinking spouts, which are certainly less messy if baby grabs the cup and tilts it. Others have heavy round bases to prevent tipping easily. It is an individual preference for you and your baby, but you should keep in mind that the cup should be unbreakable and have no sharp edges.

Between twenty-eight and thirty-two weeks, babies demonstrate the beginning of chewing patterns (up-and-down movements of the jaw); and the tongue shows more maturity during spoon-feeding. The baby can suck from a cup, but liquid often dribbles from the corners of his mouth as he projects his tongue before swallowing.

Barley: Barley contains extremely small amounts of sodium (salt) and is therefore good in a low-salt diet. Nutritionally, ¼ cup of cooked barley provides approximately 46 calories, most coming from carbohydrates. It does contain some protein, as well as thiamine, niacin, and iron. Barley is one of the oldest foods known. Wild barley was a dietary staple during some of the earliest civilizations, when a paste was made from coarse barley flour. It was then eaten fresh or dried for later use.

Late September (6½ Months)

Mirabai is sleeping now from seven or eight o'clock at night to around six A.M. or so, which is wonderful for us. It wasn't difficult, although we had to let her cry for three nights. The first night she cried strongly for about five minutes. The second night she was less vehement, and by the third night a little whimper was all we heard. And that was it. Before I put her to bed, we sit in the rocking chair and I sing lullabies while she nurses. As soon as she wakes up in the morning, I bring her into our bed and nurse her before we get up.

Some parents feel that starting solids will encourage their baby to sleep through the night. Because of this belief, some infants are started on solids as early as two months of age. Besides being inadvisable nutritionally to start solids earlier than the fifth or sixth month, research has shown that feeding solids has no apparent effect on the sleeping patterns of infants.

Early October (6½ Months)

Mirabai is now well adjusted to all the cereals and seems to look forward to her "solid meals." She also gets an egg yolk with her breakfast cereal. She doesn't care for it hard-boiled but readily accepts it soft-boiled. She eats the yolk, and I finish the white.

Today I mashed ¼ ripe banana and added it to the breakfast menu. She loved it and finished every last bit, smacking her lips and smiling. Her two bottom teeth are through and the top ones are on their way.

It is recommended that your baby be given hard-boiled egg yolk initially, as it is easier to digest. However, if he seems to prefer a soft-cooked yolk (boiled for at least 5 minutes), and seems to tolerate it well, you might try offering it that way. You should watch for reactions, however. It is wise to withhold giving the white of egg until the child is twelve months of age, since it may cause an allergic reaction. If your child has no tendency toward allergies, and there are none in your family, it should be all right to give him a whole scrambled egg, or to use a whole egg in cooking, during the latter part of the first year.

Although not as inexpensive as they used to be, bananas are still affordable and available year-round. This fruit is rich in natural fiber, high in potassium, low in sodium, and contains the vitamins A, C, and B_6 as well as thiamine, riboflavin, and niacin. Maybe out of a misconception that it is cheaper, easier, or faster to buy baby foods than make their own, many mothers will buy jars of mashed bananas. Because water is the first ingredient listed, the banana may well account for less than half of the jar's contents. Always review the labels on commercial baby foods. Ingredient information is shown in order of quantity of each ingredient. For example, the label on a jar of one manufacturer's strained bananas lists the following ingredients: water, fully ripened bananas, orange juice, sugar, tapioca starch modified, vitamin C, and citric acid. With respect to tapioca, I should mention that it is a complex starch, often difficult for an infant to digest. Most commercially prepared fruits, such as plums, bananas, and apricots, contain tapioca. It is cheaper and just as easy to mash a ripe banana, and it is certainly healthier for the baby.

Mid-October (7 Months)

I ran out of Mirabai's precooked cereal, so I made some regular oatmeal, which I gave her unsweetened with whole milk. She was hungry enough to eat half a bowlful, but certainly didn't like it as much as her baby cereal. She also had a soft-boiled egg yolk and ½ cup of apple juice with vitamin C, which she really enjoyed.

It has been suggested that parents feed their infant hot cereals fortified with iron until the child is eighteen months old. Egg yolk and infant cereals fortified with iron are good sources of this important mineral, as is regular oatmeal. The vitamin C in apple juice will help the body absorb iron.

Note: Some infant formulas are also fortified with iron, as are most infant multiple vitamins. Since some experts feel there is a danger of iron toxicity, check with your pediatrician to ensure that your baby is receiving an adequate but not excessive amount of iron.

Late October (7½ Months)

Mirabai seems to be gaining too much weight. She is not crawling yet, and until six weeks ago was nursing every four to five hours around the clock as well as getting three meals a day. Bob takes care of her on Saturdays and Sundays while I am working and I think he tends to overfeed her. He likes to snack through the day and shares whatever he eats with Mirabai. I will write breakfast, lunch, and dinner menus for him and discourage him from giving her snacks in between. Now that she is getting an adequate supply of calories, protein, fat, and carbohydrates through her daily meals, I will cut down on breast-feeding, too.

Overfeeding can be a problem in infancy. The average healthy baby from five months to one year requires 47 calories per pound of weight. (These values are given as a basic guide. Degree of activity, sleeping patterns, and the general nature of the child must be taken into consideration.) If a baby weighs 17 pounds, he should take in approximately 800 calories a day. Most formulas contain around 20 calories per ounce, breast milk containing only a fraction less. If no solids are being given, this means that a baby needs five 8-ounce feedings a day (40 ounces).

If an infant is receiving three meals a day (approximately the following meal schedule), he will have a calorie intake of 320, which leaves 480 calories for bottle or breast milk, or approximately three feedings (24 ounces). Therefore, the amount of formula or nursing should now be cut back two feedings (16 ounces).

Meal Schedule

Breakfast:	¼ cup cooked cereal		26 cal
	1 egg yolk, cooked		60 cal
	½ small banana		40 cal
		Total	126 cal
Lunch:	1 tbsp. cottage cheese		15 cal
	1 tbsp. cooked carrots		3 cal
	1 breadstick		38 cal
	3 oz. grape juice		60 cal
		Total	116 cal
Dinner:	¼ cup mashed potato		34 cal
	1 tbsp. green beans		3 cal
	½ oz. hamburger		41 cal
		Total	78 cal

Total daily intake = 320 calories solids

Early November (7½ Months)

Lunch today consisted of 2 tablespoons of spinach, 1 tablespoon of yogurt with ¼ mashed banana, and juice. I made fresh pineapple and carrot juices in the juicer and mixed a little of each in a cup for Mirabai. She took a couple of sips and then turned her head away. After being offered the rest on a spoon, she finished it off and still had a little room for some rice pudding with raisins and milk.

Following her afternoon nap, we went into the garden to enjoy the sun. It was warm but not really hot, so I took off Mirabai's clothes and watched her play with the cat and some leaves while wearing just her sun hat.

Vitamin D can be produced by the body through the action of direct sunlight on the skin. If the body is not exposed to sufficient sunlight, a dietary source of vitamin D is necessary. The best source is fish liver oils, although children often find these unpalatable. An excellent alternative source is milk fortified with vitamin D.

Second Week of November (8 Months)

My poor little one has intestinal flu, which started two nights ago with vomiting and a fever of 103°, followed by diarrhea. Yesterday the fever and vomiting had completely passed, thank heaven. I cut out most solids and have been primarily nursing Mirabai, although she ate a little rice cereal, which has a binding quality.

Today she had a loose but not liquid bowel movement; but her appetite has not returned, although she ate a little banana with plain yogurt. Later on I tried some mashed avocado but she refused it. Otherwise, she has been active and seems quite happy.

(After a week, her appetite was back to normal and she was on her regular solid foods schedule.)

When your child is sick, call your pediatrician regarding treatment, or take the baby for an examination, a diagnosis, and to find the possible cause of the illness. Babies' fevers tend to run quite high, and it is very important that they receive sufficient liquids to prevent dehydration, which could be very serious. At these times I would be flexible about giving your child bottles with juices, nighttime drinks, etc., and you could even go so far as to allow Seven-Up, melted fruit gelatine, or any clear liquids your child will accept. If he won't take them in a cup, give them in a bottle. The most important thing is to make sure he is getting plenty of liquids. When your child is well again, you can revert to the rules of no juice in bottles, no bottles in bed, and no sodas.

When diarrhea is present, it is usually wise to stop all milk products, fruits (except for bananas), and most vegetables and meats. If your baby has a fever and no appetite, don't worry about giving him solids, but do make sure he is taking enough liquids.

There is some question as to whether one should continue nursing or giving formula when an infant has diarrhea. It would probably depend on the gravity of the illness, but I feel that in most mild cases one could continue to nurse. Some experts advocate giving strained carrots, diluted with an equal part of boiled water, as carrots are high in potassium and sodium; and rice and rice water may be helpful in controlling diarrhea.

Tea should not be given to babies. The xanthines in tea stimulate and excite infants and children and in some cases cause excessive urination. This in turn aggravates the fluid imbalance.

Late November (8½ Months)

For Mirabai's lunch today I mashed half a banana and added it to a large tablespoonful of cottage cheese, a little of which she left on her plate. I have to be on guard not to insist that she finish everything—a temptation at times—and learn to recognize the first sign that tells me she has had enough. When her attention starts to wander, her mouth doesn't open wide, or she starts to play with her food, it's time to take the bowl away. If I don't, the next signs aren't so subtle. She just whams the spoon down like an auctioneer with a gavel, and there it is, baby food everywhere.

There seems to be a universal parental attitude, probably passed down through generations, that dinner isn't finished until the plate is empty. Waste is sinful. This may be true, but how can we gauge an infant's appetite? A little baby cannot tell us how hungry he is, what he enjoys eating, or when he is full. So we tend to use our own concepts of how much he needs, believing he should be full when his plate is empty. This can be when the miserable habit of overeating starts. Children have fine appetite control and react immediately when their stomachs send the message that they are full. This is very valuable in learning just how much food the body needs, and I wonder how many adults are still so well attuned.

Because your baby cannot talk, he will relay his feelings through various kinds of sign language. Each child has his own way of communicating, and parents must learn to observe the signs and respond to his needs.

Late November (8½ Months)

I have been flat on my back with the flu and a very high fever, and have been too sick to care about anything or anyone, including Mirabai. Fortunately, I have a good support system in my husband, Bob, and our two teenage sons. They have taken care of Mirabai and fed her well, and she doesn't seem to be suffering. In spite of my inability to give her any attention, and the fact that I had to stop breast-feeding abruptly, she is her usual happy self. As I had been taking lots of aspirin for the fever and was only taking liquids, I refrained from nursing her. Luckily, my breasts did not become engorged. Instead of my nursing Mirabai first thing in the morning, Bob would warm some formula when she woke up, put her in my arms, and, holding her close, I would give her the bottle. She seemed perfectly content. Although now I am well again, Mirabai has not nursed for five days, so this seems to be an appropriate time to stop. She is almost eight and a half months old, is a good weight, and the weaning did not seem to cause any trauma. Ten days later, while I was doing exercises without a bra, Mirabai started playing with my nipple. She didn't try to put it in her mouth and I knew then that she did not miss nursing and had been ready for weaning.

The time for weaning a baby is a personal choice and different circumstances may influence one's decision. Some mothers may have to return to work and would find it inconvenient to continue nursing. Others may express milk for daytime feedings and nurse only mornings and evenings.

Medical opinion is overwhelmingly in favor of breast-feeding, as it is nutritionally and psychologically better for babies. Apparently, the longer an infant can nurse, the better. However, the day will come when you have to decide to stop nursing, and a couple of factors should be kept in mind. During the nine- to twelve-month period, an infant's desire to explore his environment begins to exceed his hunger for food. His interest in bottle or breast is decreasing as the discovery of his increased motor activity becomes more important to him. This time, then, seems developmentally conducive to weaning. Solid-food eating habits also often improve after weaning because the infant is not so easily satiated by liquids.

Until the tenth to twelfth month, the average infant has relied mostly on sucking and swallowing to take his food. The ability to chew then swallow firmer foods has been progressively maturing, however, so ideally around twelve months seems like a good time to stop nursing. This would also be the time to start weaning your child from the bottle. Prolonged bottle feeding may cause two health problems. One is the bottle-mouth syndrome when severe dental cavities are caused by bed- and naptime bottles. The other is iron-deficiency anemia, caused by drinking an excessive amount of cow's milk, which contains negligible amounts of iron. (Parents concerned that thumb-sucking may be substituted for bottle feedings will be comforted to know that, as a rule, a baby who has not started thumb-sucking by eight months will generally not develop the habit thereafter.)

From about twelve to fifteen months of age, a toddler can hold and drink from a cup independently and should be able to take all his liquids this way.

One last observation on breast-feeding, which is very subjective and has not been substantiated scientifically: The hesitation of a mother to stop nursing after the first year may have more to do with the mother's psychological attachment to it than to the child's needs. There is tremendous comfort, warmth, peace, and joy in the intimacy of nursing, and often a sense of "emptiness," as well as relief, follows when breast-feeding is discontinued.

Early December (8½ Months)

Mirabai has eight teeth now (although no molars as yet) and her gag reflex is well developed. She grasps things with her hands but doesn't use her thumb and index finger yet.

I decided to try finger foods for lunch today. We started with a stoned-wheat cracker and cream cheese, which she seemed to enjoy squishing in her tiny fingers. It must have tasted good, too, for the whole thing disappeared in no time. We followed this with a little meat cake, a few pieces of cooked carrot, and a slice of peeled ripe pear, all of which were accompanied by appreciative noises. The floor was a disaster, as was the high chair, but it took no time to clean up, and when naptime came along, it was a very contented little Mirabai who went right off to sleep.

Indications that an infant is ready for finger foods are his ability to sit up, grasp and bring an object to his mouth, and the basic up-and-down chewing movements of the jaw. Initially babies grasp things with the palm of the hand, so the size and shape of finger foods are important. Start out giving him a piece of dry toast or a cracker. Once the pincer reflex is developed, the variety of finger foods offered can be increased, as your baby will be able to pick up small pieces of cooked vegetables, meat, cheese, or fruit with his thumb and index finger.

Mid-December (9 Months)

My little one's eating habits are changing and her rejection of certain foods shows her dislikes very clearly. Avocado is the most recent offender. I have tried it in combination with cottage cheese, beans, and bananas, all of which she loves, but she recognizes the avocado in all of them. The look of loathing and disgust she displays as she spits it out has made me give up this delicious fruit for the time being.

Avocado is extremely nutritious, containing at least eight essential vitamins and five vital minerals. It is high in vitamin A (carotene), folic acid, vitamin C, iron, vitamin E, and magnesium. It is an excellent source of potassium and also contains riboflavin, thiamine, pyridoxine, pantothenic acid, niacin, and choline. Its smooth texture, gentle flavor, and easy digestibility make it a desirable food for infants. Knowing this,

I tried every conceivable way to serve it to Mirabai, but for now all is in vain.

When a child exhibits a strong dislike for certain foods, this should be accepted. Foods with the same nutritional values can be substituted, although it may take several other kinds to compensate for the nutrients of the one food the baby rejects. With a little knowledge and some imagination, however, both mother and baby can win. If the rejected food is taken away and not offered again for some months, the infant's tastes may change and he may later accept it.

Variety is important to an adequate diet and a mother's challenge with a new baby is to introduce him to a large selection of nutritious foods. Problems will arise if the parents are fussy eaters. If Father won't eat certain foods, Mother usually goes out of her way not to prepare them for the rest of the family. In the same way, Mother seldom buys produce that she dislikes. In this way, rejection of many foods may be passed down from parents to children. Having a new baby around should encourage all the members of the family to examine their own eating habits.

When introducing a new food, start with a very tiny portion. The child may look at it, feel it, or just smell it initially. This is part of learning to accept it. Some children reject all foods of a certain texture, so it may help to combine a soft food with a crisp or chewy food. The color and attractiveness of food influence appetites as well. Fresh steamed broccoli, for instance, is bright green. If overcooked and left standing around, it becomes soggy and a murky green. The same is true of fresh spinach. Mix the colors of vegetables to make them more appealing; for instance, combine small pieces of cauliflower, carrots, yellow squash, and green vegetables to stimulate an unenthusiastic palate. Do not verbally reinforce your child's dislike of a food. Psychologically he may resist trying it again at a later time, even if he would like to try it.

Late December (9½ Months)

For the first time, Mirabai joined the whole family for our evening meal. I had made *får-i-kål*, a delicious Norwegian lamb and cabbage dish, which I served with potatoes boiled in their skins. Mirabai shared everything from my plate, chopped up, of course, and loved it all.

Eating together as a family group builds closeness and family solidarity. Increasingly, however, families tend not to eat together as often as they did in the past. We are becoming a society of "snackers," often eating hurriedly and alone while engaged in other activities. Sharing meals in a warm, cheerful environment can evoke in all of us positive reactions toward specific foods that go far beyond their nutritional values.

Mid-January (10 Months)

I don't know if it is her age, the irregular routine caused by our Christmas celebrations, or because she is cutting teeth—her lower lateral incisors—but Mirabai's appetite has decreased, and for the first time since she was born, she has a diaper rash. I am giving her food she is familiar with and likes, but still she takes only a few spoonfuls before spitting it out. It is frustrating and a little disconcerting, but as she sleeps soundly, has rosy cheeks, is very lively, and still seems to be gaining weight, she must be getting sufficient nutrients.

Changes in daily routine, teething, and biochemical conditions in the body that influence the acceptance of food may be among the many reasons a child's appetite decreases. Parents often worry unduly about this. If your infant is off his food but gaining weight, is active, and is sleeping well, try to relax. Children are extremely sensitive to negative as well as positive emotions, and will react to your anxiety. If no fuss is made over these periods of poor eating, the problem will resolve itself. However, if your child appears listless, loses weight, or continues to reject food for some time, you should consult your doctor. A healthy child will eat when he is hungry. If he doesn't want his meal, remove it. Don't offer alternative foods, coax, play, or use tricks to make him eat. And remember that babies' stomachs are small. One tablespoonful of each food group for each of his three meals will give adequate nutrition to a twelve-month-old.

Late January (10½ Months)

I may have found a solution to Mirabai's poor eating habits. Instead of feeding her at her normal times of eight A.M., noon, and five P.M., I wait until she seems hungry. It certainly worked last night. I warmed up some leftover lamb, cabbage, potatoes, and carrots at 6:30 P.M., and she ate a huge bowlful. This was followed by some fruit gelatine. Instead of feeding her breakfast with Bob and me at eight A.M. this morning, I waited a while. Then I gave her some natural baby food cereal that came from the health-food store, followed by a soft-boiled egg and a cup of orange juice with ¼ teaspoon brewer's yeast. Again, she ate everything readily.

It is important to remember that changes can occur in a child's eating patterns. Eating should be a pleasure as well as a necessity. Most of us don't enjoy eating if we have no appetite, especially if forced to eat. It takes keen observation and good intuition to recognize when your child is hungry and needs to eat, as opposed to waiting until he is very hungry before feeding him. Also some experts feel that "starving a child to eat" will not promote good eating patterns.

Children are normally rhythmic in their habits, so satisfying their hunger should be in tune with that rhythm. Therefore, meals should be served at the same time each day whenever possible. This may conflict with adult schedules initially, but eventually infants seem to adapt to the rest of the family's mealtimes, probably because they enjoy the social interaction.

Fatigue is often a major factor in loss of appetite. An exhausted child's appetite is seldom restored until he has had a nap or a good night's sleep.

I found brewer's yeast to be an effective appetite stimulant for Mirabai, and it is an excellent source of protein and the natural B complex vitamins. However, her pediatrician recommended only ⅛ teaspoon initially, increasing the amount slowly over several months to 1 teaspoon. If you wish to start your baby on brewer's yeast, you should talk to your doctor first.

Mid-February (11 Months)

Most of America is freezing right now while here the sun is shining and it is warm and beautiful. Mirabai and I picked camellias and irises from the garden, listened to the birds singing, and enjoyed the smell of freshly cut grass. After such a lovely time, we were more than ready for lunch. As our finances and budget have been feeling the effects of the economy, I have been using my imagination and trying to create tasty meals based on beans, rice, or pasta. I had already cooked rice and lima beans, which I reheated for lunch, with some freshly steamed broccoli. I gave Mirabai a tablespoonful of each, turned on Mahler's First Symphony, which has lots of boom-boom, and watched the rice and vegetables disappear with much banging-of-the-spoon accompaniment and laughter. Mirabai wasn't at all concerned that she was eating variations of the same foods for the second or third day. Banana with milk finished off her lunch, giving her everything she needed for a balanced meal. Before putting her down for her nap, I gave her a warm bath and a gentle massage with baby oil.

Lima beans are incomplete in protein, but combined with rice they make a complete protein, including all the essential eight amino acids. Broccoli provides a substantial amount of vitamins A and C, in addition to some calcium, iron, thiamine, riboflavin, and niacin. The banana provides more of the same, plus potassium; and milk contains calcium, protein, and vitamins A and D.

Nutritious foods do not have to be expensive. For instance, the protein in meat or fish can be substituted by the protein in beans and rice, which can be prepared in a variety of healthy and delicious ways. Vegetables and fruits that are plentiful and in season are the most economical to use along with bananas, which are available year-round and are inexpensive for the nutritional value they provide. It is also possible to keep the food budget down by utilizing cheaper cuts of meat and poultry for soups and stews, using lots of fresh vegetables, and combining incomplete proteins as shown in the table on page 25.

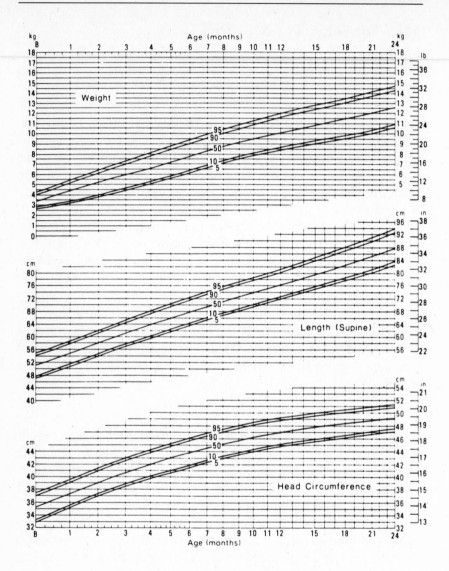

PERCENTILE STANDARDS FOR GROWTH
BOYS (BIRTH TO 24 MONTHS)

Adapted from NCHS Growth Charts

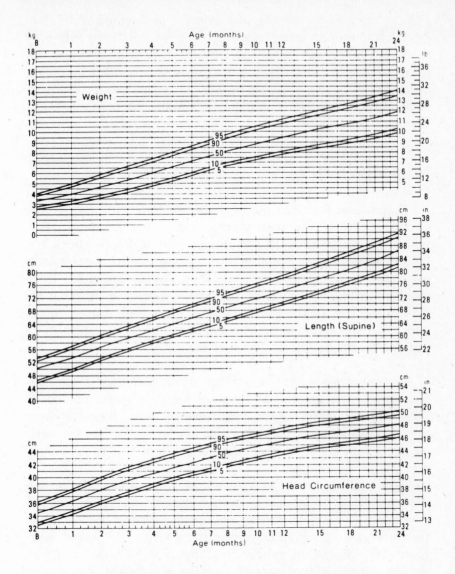

PERCENTILE STANDARDS FOR GROWTH
GIRLS (BIRTH TO 24 MONTHS)

Adapted from NCHS Growth Charts

*Many other things can give us a feeling of well-being and are abso-
lutely free: sunshine, a tree, a beautiful flower, music, or a little body
massage. Children are extremely sensitive to parental emotions and
moods, and if you are anxious, your child will be affected. With a
little conscious effort, it should be possible to turn this mood around
and make your little one's mealtimes happy and free from stress, and
allow him to enjoy his food.*

Mid-March (1 Year)

Mirabai and I visited the pediatrician today for a first-year
checkup. She is shy with strangers and became very upset
when the nurse tried to put her on the scales to check her
height and weight. Whether the measurements were totally
accurate is questionable, but they were probably close
enough. After her initial "torturous" experience, Mirabai accepted the rest of the examination with a little more compo-
sure, and she received a clean bill of health at a weight of 22
pounds and a height of 28½ inches.

*At six months of age, the average infant will have doubled his
birth weight. By his first birthday, as the child enters the toddler
phase, he will have reached approximately three times his birth
weight, stand about 29 inches tall, and have six teeth. (See the charts
on pages 110–111 for a breakdown of the first two years' growth
rates.)*

*An annual assessment of a child's weight and height gives im-
portant indicators of normal growth, as does measuring the head cir-
cumference. The most critical and rapid period of human brain
growth begins at conception and continues into the second year.
Brain cells increase in number until the child is twelve to fifteen
months of age, and they increase thereafter in mass and size. A rapid
growth in brain mass is accompanied by an increased head circumfer-
ence. Malnourished children usually have smaller head circumfer-
ences than those of their well-nourished peers. These children have
also been reported to perform more poorly on intelligence tests than
do well-nourished children. It seems that a malnourished infant has
less chance of recovering intellectual defects caused by serious nutri-*

tional deficiencies than those who become malnourished later in life. A child's ability to catch up also appears to be influenced by the length of the period of deprivation. Research has also shown that children who have been malnourished for no more than four months are less handicapped than those who have been deprived for longer periods of time.

Late March (12½ Months)

Now that Mirabai is a year old, I see a lot of changes in her. She is strong-willed and is developing a distinct personality. She insists on feeding herself and has become very opinionated about what she will eat. If what she is being served doesn't please her, even without so much as a taste, she turns ninety degrees in her high chair, shakes her head vigorously, and clamps her mouth shut. And there is no consistency to this young lady's likes and dislikes. She may accept something today that she refused yesterday and may refuse again tomorrow. While she wants to use a spoon, it is purely accidental and quite miraculous if she scoops up any food, as she plunges the spoon into her bowl impatiently and usually turns it upside down before it reaches her mouth. Most of a meal ends up outside her body, on the floor, and covering the high chair. If she is very hungry, I am allowed to guide her hand with the spoon, and we might get a couple of spoonsful of food into her mouth. Otherwise, it's back to finger feeding.

This is a very trying time indeed. It calls for tremendous patience and understanding, but it is important not to discourage this independence. Self-feeding is one of a child's first steps toward independence and controlling his environment. The learning process can be frustrating at this age because motor skills are not sufficiently developed, so a mother's role becomes that of teacher. Show your child how to hold a spoon, gently bringing his hand to his mouth, and he will eventually get the necessary movements under control. It can be a long, slow process, since children tend to fluctuate between resis-

*tance and cooperation, but your efforts will be rewarded when your
toddler shows you "I can do it all by myself."*

*Last, as left- or right-handed dominance has not been established
and should not be enforced, allow your child to grab the spoon with
either hand. In another three or four months, finer control of the
wrist and fingers will be established and self-feeding will be considerably more efficient and speedy.*

Early April (12½ Months)

I occasionally give Mirabai a dried apricot for a snack or
treat. Since she has no molars, she mostly gums the fruit,
working on it for quite a while. She takes it out of her mouth,
examines it, pops it back in, and generally seems to enjoy the
taste and experience. However, the apricot comes out whole
in her bowel movements as do whole corn kernels. Obviously
she is not able to chew them up. Fortunately, Mirabai has
never choked on food. I am very careful to mash or finely cut
her food because, even though she has a few teeth, she
doesn't seem to take the time to chew her food.

*The problem of toddlers and small children choking on food became
alarm enough for the federal government to appoint a national task
force to study the problem. Results showed that hundreds of children
have died from choking on food, with hot dogs and grapes being the
biggest offenders. Always keep in mind that toddlers and small children often do not chew food thoroughly, so consider not giving them
potential choke foods until they are older.*

*Some potential choke foods are peanuts and other nuts, whole corn,
grapes, cherries, whole orange segments (with membranes), raw
whole carrots, and hot dogs.*

Late April (13½ Months)

Last week for dinner I gave Mirabai mashed potatoes and
carrots, followed by cottage cheese and cantaloupe, and she
ate it all. When I tried the same foods today, she wouldn't

touch them. I am concerned that if I try to coax her with alternative foods I may be encouraging finicky eating habits. Her two teenage brothers, who believe they are authorities on child rearing because they have just outgrown childhood themselves, knew exactly what to do and shared such wisdom as "If she doesn't want it, take the food away," and "Don't give her anything else to eat until she finishes what she has." Then they watch while, with an uneasy mind, I pick Mirabai up and put her to bed without any dinner.

I do believe in consistency and discipline, but it is sometimes difficult to follow through and I wonder if I am doing the right thing. The boys' absolute assurance on the subject annoys me, and I point out to William his problem with eating beans and many vegetables. He quickly answers that that is exactly the point; he doesn't want us to make the same mistakes with Mirabai that were made with him! This is a subject continually being raised by both boys, who feel we should have been more strict and consistent with them. Mirabai has always received a lot of attention, but if she cries for something she can't have, she is totally ignored, and she has never thrown a tantrum because she wasn't allowed a cookie, candy, or toy that caught her fancy. She may cry out of frustration for a while, then everything is fine again. Persistent angry tears have never given her good results, and this makes everyone's life much easier.

Discipline is a very important part of a child's life and is necessary in establishing good eating habits. However, it is not always easy to enforce, especially when one is anxious that a child has not had enough to eat. We are vulnerable and open to manipulation, and children are remarkably astute at using this advantage. It is important to be consistent without being authoritarian, stubborn, punitive, or angry.

Early May (13½ Months)

Mirabai is having regular oatmeal with milk for breakfast. She has a spoon and I am sitting watching her. Although the spoon is used only occasionally, she is eating happily and en-

eing the oatmeal squeeze through her little fingers she makes a fist. There is oatmeal splattered on the walls, and the floor and high chair are covered. Mirabai is having a wonderful time. I am not. It is difficult to watch her, and I want to take the bowl and spoon and feed her myself—neat, clean, and easy. She will not learn to feed herself if I do, but at what point should I intervene? It is important and natural for toddlers to touch food. Using fingers is acceptable for certain foods, and a toddler is not yet able to distinguish between those that may be handled and those that may not, and why. Nor does neatness count. However, this is the time to start learning. I don't want Mirabai to think she is bad, dirty, or naughty because she is touching her food or making a mess, but when she loses interest in using the spoon altogether, I take it from her and feed her myself. If she refuses to give up her spoon, I get another one and use that. When she is full, I remove the bowl immediately so that leftovers can't be used as playthings.

One day I gave Mirabai her spoon and some yogurt in a bowl. Apparently she couldn't eat it fast enough with a spoon, and fingers were of no use, so before I realized what was happening, she picked up the bowl and had yogurt trickling down her face, dress, chair, and the floor. It was a terrible mess but I had to laugh.

Parents should understand that children in this age group need some freedom to experiment in order to assert independence. If a toddler is to master new skills, he must have adult approval of his trials-and-errors in learning.

"Shaping" and "fading" are two techniques professionals use to teach self-feeding. Shaping is the reinforcement of each step needed for the task to be learned. The first step is taught, then reinforced, and when it is learned, the next step is added and reinforced. This pattern continues until the desired behavior is obtained. An example of teaching spoon feeding by shaping works in the following way:

Step 1: Child looks at spoon.
Step 2: Child moves hand toward spoon.
Step 3: Child touches spoon.

Step 4: Child picks up spoon.
Step 5: Child puts spoon in dish.
Step 6: Child scoops up food.
Step 7: Child brings food to mouth.
Step 8: Child takes food off spoon.
Step 9: Child returns spoon to dish.
Reinforcement = Bites of food or praise as each step is accomplished.

Fading offers a different approach. Instead of requiring the child to proceed through several steps, the trainer's cues are changed as the child's skills develop. For example, the trainer holds the child's hand around a spoon and puts him through the motions of scooping food into it, bringing the spoon to his mouth, and returning the spoon to the dish. As the child gradually assumes independent movement, physical assistance is decreased, and the trainer provides help only when needed to complete the task.

Most parents use these techniques instinctively in teaching their children self-feeding, but the psychological definitions of shaping and fading may clarify the steps and help parents work through this difficult stage more easily.*

Mid-May (14 Months)

The skies have been overcast for weeks, but today there is a gentle breeze, the sun is shining, and at last it feels like summer. After Mirabai's morning nap, we decided to have a picnic lunch in the garden. Mirabai ran around dressed only in a little sun hat while I spread a blanket under the apricot tree and brought out a tray with wheat crackers, Swiss cheese, and grape juice for us. After enjoying this light but satisfying lunch, Mirabai played with the cat while I wrote a letter. Although I hadn't intended to stay outside too long, two hours passed in a wink and I decided to give Mirabai a cooling bath. After some bathtub play and a little baby-oil massage, we

*Source: *Nutrition in Infancy and Childhood*, Peggy L. Pipes, The C. V. Mosby Company, St. Louis, Mo., 1977.

snacked on some leftover white beans, cottage cheese, and watermelon. Mirabai fed herself, getting almost as many beans on herself and the floor as in her tummy, which made me realize I should have waited for the bath. But she is trying hard to use the spoon and is learning. If I were a little braver and let her eat everything independently, she would probably become adept very quickly.

In warmer weather it is wise to serve lighter meals, with a greater emphasis on fruits and cheese, foods that don't require cooking and are nutritious, refreshing, and easily digested.

Cheese is a concentrated source of many of the nutrients found in milk. It is an excellent source of protein and calcium, contributes significant amounts of phosphorus and riboflavin to the diet, and contains vitamin B_{12} and magnesium. Its high-quality protein, vitamins, and minerals make it a very valuable food. Milk and dairy products are the richest source of calcium in the North American diet, and the recommended daily requirement is 800 milligrams for a one- to three-year-old child.

Mozzarella, jack, Swiss (Jarlsberg), Cheddar, and Bel Paese cheeses are good to use for finger foods. Parmesan cheese has a strong flavor but is very rich in protein, so let your child eat it if he likes it. All types of cottage cheese are good and blend well with fruits. Ricotta is a creamy Italian cheese used mostly in cooking, but it can be served with fruit as well. It has a higher fat content than cottage cheese and is an excellent source of calcium.

Another benefit from cheese has recently been found. Charles Schachtele, an oral microbiologist, made some interesting discoveries when measuring the impact of cheese on teeth. Swiss, jack, and aged Cheddar cheeses were found to be very effective in blocking formation of the acid that can cause tooth decay. Blue, Brie, Gouda, and mozzarella cheeses are not as effective, but they still inhibit tooth decay. The least effective cheeses in retarding acid buildup are feta, provolone, cream cheese, and all processed cheeses.

Toddlers need to be encouraged to feed themselves, progressing from finger foods to utensils. Eating is a sensual experience for a young child and one must expect messiness in self-feeding. Parents should be encouraged to allow the child to develop independence in this as soon as he is ready.

Late May (14½ Months)

We had Chinese food for dinner last night. I stir-fried some boned cut-up chicken in the wok with bean sprouts, mushrooms, onions, and snow peas, and served them with basmati rice. Mirabai ate very little, as she had had a late lunch and was obviously not very hungry. I should have taken her cue. She has well-regulated eating habits, does not eat for the sake of it, and I never force food on her. However, we were having strawberries and kiwi fruit for dessert, which she loves, so I gave her some. The colors of the fruit appealed to her and she stuffed them into her mouth as fast as she could, with obvious pleasure. Later that night everything came back up, poor little one. But I needn't have worried, for when she woke up this morning, she was chirpy as ever and ready for breakfast.

Recently Mirabai threw back her head to laugh and I noticed that two upper molars had broken through. Besides a slight decline in appetite, some drooling, and putting her fingers in her mouth, she showed no problems. I had worried that she would have a difficult time cutting the molars, as her gums were so swollen and looked painful, but obviously they didn't bother her.

The time when teeth are cut varies greatly from child to child. The following schedule gives the approximate time deciduous teeth (baby teeth) should show through:

- Lower central incisors (2): 5–9 months
- Upper central incisors (2): 8–12 months
- Upper lateral incisors (2): 10–12 months
- Lower lateral incisors (2): 12–15 months
- First molars (4): 10–16 months
- Canines (4): 16–20 months
- Second molars (4): 20–30 months

The average child will have six teeth at one year of age, twelve teeth at eighteen months, sixteen teeth at two years, and twenty teeth at two and a half years.

Although all children's reactions differ, teething will present problems and changes in their daily lives to some degree. Doctors feel that teething does not cause fever, diarrhea, or a runny nose. However, these symptoms seem to appear with teething almost universally. A baby may develop diaper rash for the first time, be cranky and irritable, or suffer from loss of appetite. Since so many teeth are being cut during the first two years, there will be many trying times. On the positive side, children seem to bounce back remarkably quickly from whatever symptoms they had; a high fever and no appetite for several days may be all but forgotten within a week. If your child has a fever, check with your pediatrician first and give the child plenty of liquids. It is important to get the fever down as soon as possible. Should your baby have diarrhea, cut out fruits, milk, and milk products until the symptoms have disappeared. Plain boiled rice or rice water can be helpful in stopping diarrhea. Diaper rash should be kept to a minimum by changing your child as soon as he becomes wet or soiled. A mixture of Desitin and A & D Ointment makes a soothing skin barrier. Fresh air and a little sunshine also promote healing.

Teething is a troublesome time for parents as well as baby. Extra love, patience, attention, and cuddling are needed. Don't be concerned that your child will become a hypochondriac if you give him unlimited attention and love while he is feeling so bad. If you give him the love he needs when he is well, extra care during an illness will have no negative long-term effects. If times of illness are the only times a child gets special consideration, love, and attention, this may cause a future problem.

Mid-June (15 Months)

Mirabai and I went for a long walk today. I put her in the stroller and we went to the shopping mall, mainly to window-shop. We hadn't had lunch and were hungry, so I looked for a place to eat. A hot dog from the fast-food stand was outrageously expensive for a puny-looking wiener on a dry white bun. The hamburgers didn't look any better, so we went to the health-food store and bought some Bulgarian yogurt with raspberries in the bottom, a small carton of milk, and a peach, all of which Mirabai and I shared. We sat on a bench in the sun and watched the people pass by. Little sparrows came hopping up to us, looking for crumbs, so next time we come on this small adventure, we will bring some crackers or bread so Mirabai can feed the birds as well as herself.

Taking children shopping is usually a necessity, seldom a pleasure. Little ones get bored and restless very easily, and often by the time the parent decides to stop for a snack or lunch, they are too tired to eat. One of the most common reasons for poor appetite is fatigue, so it is wise not to wait too long before stopping for a break. Both mother and child will benefit in the long run.

Sitting in a chair for any length of time is very trying for a child, and there are usually alternatives to going to restaurants and coffee shops. If the weather is good, look for a park, a small grassy area, or even a bench, and have a minipicnic. Either bring food or buy what you need at the store. Cheese and crackers, fruit, and milk or juice will be plenty for a shopping luncheon. Occasionally, of course, the whole family may decide to go to a restaurant, and this requires a little more forethought. If your baby is very young and eating puréed or mashed foods, take a small food mill with you. Any vegetable, meat, or starch can be turned into baby food, but keep in mind that the restaurant food will probably contain quite a bit of salt (although I don't feel an occasional meal with salt will be harmful). As the baby grows older, he will be able to share the restaurant meal with you. The main concern is how to keep him entertained while you wait for dinner. A story, simple puzzle, or toy will keep a toddler occupied, but your attention and participation will be needed. Expecting a small child to entertain himself will probably not work.

Late June (15½ Months)

A few weeks ago I attended a cooking demonstration by Marion Cunningham (editor of *The Fannie Farmer Cookbook*). She made breads and a fresh fruit soup. Many fruit soups originated in Scandinavia and making this one in class brought back memories. My mother's recipe was made with blueberries picked from the mountain slopes by my father. She mixed the berries with water, sugar, and a little potato flour (to thicken). After bringing the mixture to a boil and cooking it for a few minutes, she would cool it and serve it for dessert with a dollop of whipped cream. Similar soups were made with apples, rhubarb, or rosehips, and oats, semolina, or rye would sometimes be added. It was a very nutritious dessert. Mrs. Cunningham's soup called for fresh strawberries, a little sugar, yogurt, a dash of Grand Marnier, and fresh mint, mixed well in the blender. It was delicious.

It has been very hot recently, so I thought it would be a pleasant dessert to try on my family, leaving out the Grand Marnier for Mirabai's sake, and using homemade yogurt. It tasted good, and I refrigerated it for several hours so that it would be well chilled. On opening the refrigerator to serve my new specialty, I was amazed to find only 4 tablespoonsful left. I gave what little there was to Bob and Mirabai, who loved it. The mystery of the disappearing fruit soup was cleared up when my eldest son, William, came home and complimented me on the great strawberry smoothie I had made! A couple of days later I tried again. This time everyone shared it and Mirabai ate a whole bowlful.

We are more familiar with hot soups, made with meat and vegetables, than with cold fruit soups. However, this is a truly delicious way of encouraging your family to eat yogurt and fresh fruit. Strawberries are an excellent source of vitamin C, and yogurt makes a good substitute for a serving of milk.

Fourth of July (15½ Months)

It would have been nice to go to the beach on this hot Independence Day, but the freeways and beaches are so crowded that we are content to celebrate at home. A lot of friends and their children are coming over for a potluck party. One family is bringing potato salad, another a green salad, and someone else the buns and paper goods; and we are going to barbecue the traditional hot dogs and hamburgers and make homemade ice cream. The kids will have fresh lemonade using lemons from the garden, and the grown-ups can also have beer or wine.

The garden is full of laughter, talk, and the occasional scream of excitement from one of the little ones. The ice-cream machine is churning away, the barbecue has stopped smoking, and Bob is expertly cooking the meat and corn. Mirabai is in her element. She loves parties. Right now she is sitting under the apricot tree with Grandma, balancing a paper plate on her little knees and tasting all the different foods, while her little friend Robert is cleaning up everyone's plate, whether they have finished or not. Maybe the relaxed atmosphere, sunshine, and wonderful company have something to do with it, but everything we ate tasted so delicious, and now we are waiting for the grand finale, the homemade ice cream. There is nothing in the world so good as do-it-yourself ice cream, even if it is a little soft, and it disappears in no time. Everyone helps with the cleaning up, and as the sun is setting, the little ones are getting sleepy. Mirabai doesn't protest when I tuck her into bed. It has been a very special and happy day.

There are few foods as typically American—and enjoyed by so many people—as hot dogs and hamburgers. Recently, however, the nutritional value of the hot dog has come under attack. The ingredients listed on a typical pack of wieners read as follows: pork, water, beef, salt, corn syrup, dextrose, flavoring, sodium ascorbate, sodium nitrate. Which makes this food something to avoid serving to toddlers or children—or adults for that matter—on a regular basis. But sometimes the hot dog typifies a special occasion, such as the Fourth of July or a baseball game, and if the occasions are fairly infrequent, the sentimental value can override the nutritional one. I feel this also applies to cookies and candies, which should be allowed only on special occasions.

The following is an excerpt taken from a condensed Consumer Reports *article dated May 1980:*

Hot dogs are not overly nutritious. They are cheap, but high in fat. Like all cured meats they contain small amounts of nitrite or nitrate. Nitrite gives cured meat its characteristic flavor and color and inhibits the growth of bacteria, including the source of botulism, toxin. However, nitrite may combine with amines (natural compounds found in most foods) to form nitrosamines, which cause cancer in animals. The amounts of nitrites and nitrosamines in cured meats have been reduced in recent years, but nitrite is still added to foods because there is as yet no suitable substitute for it as an inhibitor of botulism. Some hot dogs are nitrite free and contain no preservatives. They must be kept frozen until cooked.

Nitrosamines are also a normal by-product of the bacteria that live in the digestive tract. We appear to have learned to live with low levels of them. Researchers state that fiber lowers the concentration of nitrosamines by increasing the size and frequency of stools and speeding their elimination from the system. The message is to cut down on fats and meats in our diet, and increase fiber through eating fruits, whole grains, and vegetables.*

Mid-July (16 Months)

I had an interesting conversation with a friend yesterday on the advantages and disadvantages of meat in babies' diets. She had read a book specifically mentioning the dangers of a vegetarian diet for babies and the possibility that this could cause deformities and deficiencies in bone structure. Such things could happen if an infant was kept on an extreme vegetarian diet excluding milk products and eggs, and if the parents lacked knowledge of how to combine incomplete proteins to make them complete.

I have mixed feelings about meat and realize I serve it much less frequently now than I did ten years ago. In the past there was a lot of controversy about livestock being injected with stilbestrol (a hormone used to promote growth) and antibiotics, so I decided to call the U.S. Department of Agriculture to get the facts. I spoke with two meat inspectors, a supervisor, and a veterinarian who works with livestock. Each reassured me that stilbestrol has now been federally outlawed. All animals are vaccinated when young to prevent a variety of diseases, in much the same way that babies are vaccinated against human diseases. Also poultry are given antibiotics of which all traces should be gone by the time they are slaughtered. All meats and poultry are checked randomly, and if any contamination is found, that meat is not made available for public consumption. That was good to hear.

More and more Americans are reducing their intake of meat, sometimes for financial reasons, sometimes for their health. Although all processed meats, such as ham, bacon, sausage, and luncheon meats, contain additives, increased consumer awareness has had a beneficial influence on the meat production industry.

If any kind of vegetarian diet is contemplated for an infant, it is extremely important that it be done with a complete understanding of how to provide total nutrition. It cannot be emphasized enough that one should not put babies on a vegetarian diet without first reading as much qualified literature as possible and becoming aware of the knowledge that must be gained before starting such a diet.

Early August (16½ Months)

I have heard so much about the nutritional value of tofu that I bought a pack today. I cubed it and sautéed it with onions and mushrooms, and served some to Mirabai with steamed broccoli and carrots. She seemed to enjoy it far more than Bob or I did. The texture was unappealing to us and the flavor was bland, but as it is healthful and inexpensive, I will experiment and incorporate it occasionally into our meals, especially since Mirabai likes it. This will also be an incentive for us to break down a few food prejudices and expand our dietary horizons.

Tofu is made from soybeans. It is rich in usable protein, contains all eight essential amino acids, and delivers more than 35 percent of its calories in the form of protein. Tofu is low in saturated fats and carbohydrates, and has no cholesterol, preservatives, coloring, or ad-

*ditives. The little fat there is contains large amounts of lecithin and
an important nutrient, linoleic acid. Besides being a good source of
calcium and other minerals, such as iron, phosphorus, and potassium, tofu also has essential B vitamins, choline, and the fat-
soluble vitamin E. Tofu is soft, very easily digested, and an excellent
food for babies.*

*Like yogurt or cottage cheese, tofu is ready to eat and requires no
preparation. However, it is extremely versatile in cooking, and can
be steamed, microwaved, broiled, sautéed, toasted, or baked. Tofu can
also be sliced, cubed, mashed, puréed, frozen, dried, or blended. Since
it is almost tasteless, it mixes well with virtually any other ingredient and will pick up the flavor and aroma of whatever it is combined
with.*

Mid-August (17 Months)

It has been so hot that Mirabai has had very little appetite
and is surviving primarily on milk, juices, and fruit. The
mornings are still fairly cool and she has a substantial breakfast, but at lunch and dinner she eats only a little before hand-
ing me her plate, saying firmly, "Away." I realize she has
picked up the habit of removing her bowl, cup, or anything
else on her tray, as this is something I do immediately when
she has had enough. But it is a habit that I encouraged totally
unconsciously.

Last week I gave Mirabai beets for lunch. Although she was
very hungry, the taste and texture did not appeal to her and
she wouldn't eat them. Looking around, she saw a banana in
the fruit basket and indicated that she wanted it. I put some
slices in her bowl and watched her alternate quite independently between the beets and banana until they all had disappeared.

*Developing independence, which starts at about nine months of
age, can be either exciting or distressing to parents. Behavior patterns may already have been formed, and from that time on, the infant will start to display them.*

During the first year an infant has tremendous adjustments to make, including adapting to new foods and methods of eating. Rebellion against unfamiliar foods can be lessened and long-term refusals prevented if parents learn to recognize their children's eating patterns. For instance, the realization that an eighteen-month-old may have a sporadic appetite, and that this is no cause for undue alarm, may prevent long-lasting battles over food.

Very hot weather may cause smaller appetites. At these times, meals should be kept light. Use tuna, cheese, eggs, and other dishes that are light and easy to prepare and work well in salads. A variety of fresh fruits and vegetables can provide sufficient vitamins and minerals, especially when they are supplemented with fruit juices and milk. Fresh fruit-juice popsicles can be made in your freezer for a healthy and refreshing treat, as well as shakes made with berries, yogurt, juices, milk, and/or ice cream.

Mid-September (18 Months)

Mirabai's vocabulary is expanding, walking has brought new-found freedom, and her feelings of self-confidence and independence are developing rapidly. I usually let her decide what she will eat for breakfast, and her choices so far have been reasonable. This morning she asked for cottage cheese, prunes, and banana with milk, and at lunchtime I gave her an egg, whole bread, fresh steamed vegetables, and fresh fruit. She is eating less than she used to and is completely independent with feeding, countering any offers of assistance with "Bibai do it." She accepts a wide variety of foods, is healthy, and generally seems to be a contented child.

I feel she is now mentally and physically mature enough to understand some simple table manners. We add the word "Please" after each request she makes and "Thank you" when she receives what she has asked for. To my delight, everyone has become very polite at mealtimes, with pleases and thank-yous everywhere. Bob and the boys have always teased me about my insistence on good manners and what they consider to be my "bourgeois pretentiousness." That is, until now. Suddenly it has become very important that Mirabai be polite and learn "correct" table manners. So we have also added

"Don't play with your food" and "Don't talk with your mouth full." These are enough rules for now, except that we always wash our hands before eating.

As Mirabai matures, we will add to her list of basic table manners: No elbows on the table, no licking fingers or knives, learning how to use utensils, and using a napkin instead of her hand to wipe her mouth.

This is a perfect opportunity for all of us to take a refresher course on our own table manners and to remember that children learn best by good example.

After the rapid development of the first year, the rate of growth slows down. Important muscle development takes place as the child learns to walk. His major back, thigh, and buttock muscles must be strengthened for walking and erect posture. Bones begin to lengthen, and more of the body's mineral deposits are used to strengthen bones to carry the extra weight.

The child has an increasing sense of self, or ego, of being a distinct individual, and starts to realize that he is not just an extension of his mother. He wants to decide and act for himself, whether he is capable of doing so or not. It is important for the parent to understand two principles at this time: (1) The child is striving for autonomy and his attempts often take the form of refusing food and wanting to be independent before he is able to be. Support and encouragement should be given in self-feeding and selection of foods. The parent should maintain a calm, relaxed attitude and express a sympathetic interest in the toddler's efforts. Give help when needed, but avoid overprotection or excessive rigidity. (2) The child needs fewer calories but more protein and minerals for growth. A variety of healthy foods should be offered in smaller quantities to provide these nutrients.

By the time a child is eighteen months old, ritual becomes very important. Acts performed the same way several times will be repeated diligently by your child, and this can offer a marvelous opportunity to establish positive habits. Young children copy everything adults do, for better or worse. Although this is a very effective way to teach children, parents may be surprised at some of the mirror images they receive of themselves. We can learn from children, as they can learn from us. These challenging times can be a positive experience for everyone.

Late September (18½ Months)

Although it was a long, hot summer, we never seemed to find time to go to the beach. With Mirabai napping at noon, there was not enough time in the mornings, and it was too late to pack up and go after her nap. But somehow I couldn't let a whole summer pass without at least one trip to the beach, so, nap or no nap, we did it today. The children are back at school, so the beaches were not crowded, and the day was clear and sunny.

I packed a simple lunch for us both with two hard-boiled eggs, one quartered tomato, whole wheat crackers, Jarlsberg cheese cubes, apple juice, and a bowl of cut-up cantaloupe and watermelon. Several changes of clothes (including a long-sleeved top and a sun hat), blanket, towel, sun-block cream, and shovel and pail were crammed into a huge straw bag, and with Mirabai, ice chest, and accessories, we set off. Mirabai fell asleep almost immediately and although it was a short nap, it seemed to be sufficient. As soon as we were settled on the sand, I gave her a liberal coating of sun-block cream and she set off to catch seagulls. Although her enthusiasm never flagged, it took her too far from our spot on the beach, and I had to watch her constantly and bring her back to "home base." All this running made her thirsty and gave her a wonderful appetite, so she really enjoyed her somewhat sandy egg, melon, and crackers. Although it was not exactly a restful day for Mamma, it was lovely to see her enjoying the freedom, and her happiness exhilarated me, too. A couple of hours or so was just enough time for this delightful new experience, and a tired little girl finished her nap on the way home.

An outing or a trip can be a mixed pleasure for parents. Once a child starts walking, he is going to get into everything possible, and

*even some things that seem impossible. The days of long adult con-
versations, reading, a serious game of chess or volleyball at the beach,
are over for a while. The focus has to shift to your little one, to
sharing his activities, explorations, and pleasures. All children love
the beach, parks, or mountains, and picnicking can be the highlight
of the day. It is as easy to prepare a nutritious picnic with yogurt,
fruit, juices, hard cheese, hard-boiled eggs, and crackers as it is to
pack potato chips, sodas, cakes, and processed cheese. Raw vegetables
with pita bread, breadsticks and homemade dip, pineapple spears,
dried apricots and peaches, and so on, will satisfy the cravings of
the fussiest appetite and the sweetest tooth, with the added bonus of
providing more fiber, vitamins, minerals, and lower calories than almost any processed food.*

*Small jars or bottles can be filled with fresh lemonade, orange,
grape, or apple juice and put in the freezer the night before an outing.
By the time you arrive at your destination you will have either fruit
slushes or icy cold drinks, depending on how far you are traveling
and how hot the weather is. A little more thought may be necessary
to prepare fresh foods than to open a bag of cookies or potato chips,
but the benefits to your child's health—to say nothing of the good
eating habits that are encouraged—make it well worthwhile.*

Mid-October (19 Months)

I had enjoyed Marion Cunningham's cooking class so much
that I decided to try another on bread making. Although I
have made bread several times, I have never been very satisfied with the results, so I hoped to find out some trade se-
crets. Today I decided to put my newfound knowledge to the
test and I baked her Health Bread (see page 249). It turned
out beautifully—light, tasty, and with a good crust—and I felt
very pleased with myself.

Mirabai loves bread and butter but always leaves the crust.
She certainly has enough teeth to handle crust, so I refuse to
trim it off in hopes that one day she will discover that that is
the best part of a loaf. She and I are the only ones in the
family who prefer whole-grain breads, as Bob's favorites are

French and Italian breads, and William swears by the ul-
trawhite, sponge-soft kind. However, when I serve home-
baked bread, everyone loves it.

*Bread is a staple food in many cultures around the world. It is
made in a vast variety of shapes and sizes with equally various grains
and flours: East Indian chapatis, Middle Eastern pita bread, Mexican tortillas, and Norwegian lefse, to mention a few—all of these
are flat unleavened breads made from wheat, corn, or potatoes.
Through the ages, different breads were made for various classes of
people, with white bread being reserved solely for the nobility.*

*White bread achieves its fine texture through the bran and germ
being removed from the wheat, which reduces its value as a food
source. Since 1970, sales of white "enriched" bread have been
dropping, and there is a growing awareness that whole-grain
breads offer more nutritional value than fortified white bread. The
kernel of the wheat plant has an outer layer, the bran, which
contains the germ and endosperm. Bran is composed of starch,
protein, oil, cellulose, fiber, minerals such as calcium and iron,
and vitamins E and the B complex. When the bran and wheat
germ are removed from white flour, many nutrients are removed
with them. To make this flour even whiter and longer lasting, it
is then bleached. Some millers replace the lost vitamins and minerals with synthetic nutrients, although the bran is not restored.
Bran is valuable for its fiber, an element that is undesirably low
in the American diet. Lack of fiber in nutrition has been linked
to diseases such as diverticulitis, obesity, gallstones, heart disease,
colorectal cancer, polyps, and hiatus hernia.*

*With more public awareness of good nutrition, millers and bakers
are adapting to the demand for a variety of whole wheat breads and
unbleached white flour, as well as stone-ground whole wheat flour.
Other flours for use in bread making (some alone, some combined
with wheat) are graham, rye, oat, barley, buckwheat, corn, soy, rice,
bran, millet, gluten, and potato. It is no longer difficult to buy good,
healthful bread in America. Should you have time to make your own,
however, you will not only get all the nutrients you want but also
discover how delicious bread can really be.*

Late October—Halloween (19½ Months)

It is Halloween, the most dreaded day of the year for me, not because of the "tricks" but because of the "treats." When my sons were children, they would return from trick-or-treating with pillowcases full of candy. Although I was able to appeal to their noble side and persuade them to give most of it to Children's Hospital, it is a custom I prefer not to start with Mirabai. So I have been dreaming up different ways of celebrating Halloween without the emphasis on candy. I bought little packages of roasted peanuts and raisins for children who come to the house, as well as three pumpkins which Robert and William have carved into lanterns. I also roasted the pumpkin seeds as treats for ourselves. Mirabai is fascinated by the children in their costumes and enjoys helping me hand out the nuts and raisins.

I realize that Halloween is a very exciting time for children, so I will try to come up with something special next year, possibly a Halloween-at-Home party with some little friends. We can make puppets, witches, ghosts and goblins, tell the tale of Halloween, and visit a few close neighbors for trick or treat. Unfortunately, today there are many psychotic people in our society who tamper with the candy or fruit they hand out, and it is essential that parents check their children's treats carefully. Unless given by friends or neighbors who are personally known to the family, any treat that is not factory sealed should be discarded.

Next year I will make Mirabai a costume, and as she grows older, we may get into the tradition of fortune telling. I am sure she will have her own ideas, too. One day I may even look forward to Halloween instead of dreading it.

Halloween, or All Hallows Eve, bears little resemblance today to its point of origin, the Celtic new year's eve, a Druid ritual of fire and remembrance of the dead through the worship of the pagan god Samhain. Bonfires were lit to help the dying sun, whose rays grew feeble at this time of year, when the human psyche was at its lowest. Through dance, meditation, and chanting, witches believed they were able to renew their physical energy and psychic forces. These rituals were later adapted to Christian ceremonies, becoming feasts in honor of all saints, All Hallows. Elves, fairies, and witches (who sometimes took the shape of cats) were believed to fly on All Hallows Eve, and large bonfires were set to ward off these spirits. Halloween was also thought to be the most favorable time for fortune telling, and apples and nuts were used for this purpose.

Irish and Scottish immigrants brought Halloween traditions with them to the United States during the late nineteenth century. In this country, a pumpkin replaced the turnip or potato used for carving jack-o'-lanterns. Bobbing for apples in a pail of water replaced their use in fortune telling. The Irish believed that "the little people" play pranks during Halloween; this started the custom of boys and men playing practical jokes on that night.

With children today wearing costumes and going from door to door to trick-or-treat, some safety measures should be kept in mind. Encourage the use of light-colored costumes, or sew on reflecting tape front and back, so the children can be easily seen by motorists. If costumes are homemade, purchase only flame-retardant material. As masks may block a child's vision, use makeup to paint a mask on his face, or at least enlarge the eye apertures in the mask to ensure maximum vision. Young trick-or-treaters should always be accompanied by an adult and carry a flashlight after dusk.

Mid-November (20 Months)

The Norwegian Seamen's Church is having its annual Christmas Bazaar this week. It is so far away from where we live, I visit only once a year, usually at the holiday season. Close to the church is a Norwegian import store, so I also stock up on all the traditional foods that are a part of our Christmas celebrations. This year we decided to pick up Bob from work and drive down to the church in the late afternoon. Mirabai took a long nap, and as she did not have time to eat before we left, I made up some little individual food bags for the long journey. One bag contained a peeled and quartered pear, another several stoned-wheat crackers, a third had two quarters of a tomato, and the last contained three small cubes of Swiss cheese. A child's vacuum flask, the kind that has a little spout, was filled with milk so that Mirabai could drink by herself without spilling.

Having lost my way to Bob's office, I was then relieved of the driving by an anxious father. By this time Mirabai was hungry, so I gave her the little bags, one at a time, which she thought was fun and enjoyed opening. After finishing everything, she sat happily and quietly for the rest of the journey.

When we arrived at the church, we found a wonderful *smøgåsasbord* of the most delicious open-faced sandwiches imaginable. They included hard-boiled eggs with anchovies, lox and scrambled eggs, *karbonade* (a kind of meat cake) with fried onions, pâté with beets and cucumber, and lots more. Mirabai was full and not at all interested, so I ate for both of us, but she did taste my *bløtkake* (sponge cake with fresh fruit and whipped cream), which is irresistible even if the tummy is full.

Traveling with children can be enjoyable and memorable. Without careful planning and consideration, however, it can also be a disaster. What is needed for a journey depends on the length of the trip, the age of your children, and the type of transportation. Some general rules apply, regardless of certain specifics.

For each child it is easiest to have a large bag containing the following:
- *A complete change of clothing, extra diapers, wet towelettes, facial tissues, and a warm sweater or coat.*
- *Individual bags containing simple foods that will not spoil, are easy to consume, and are usually enjoyed by the child. Raw or cooked vegetables and fruits, hard cheeses, crackers, or toast are good basics. Juice, milk, and water should be taken in vacuum flasks. Prefrozen cans of juice are handy if the weather is very warm. Bottles with disposable liners are good for infants on trips, as there is no need to sterilize bottles.*
- *A variety of toys in simple containers such as plastic bowls with lids or a cloth drawstring bag, keeping in mind your child's age and limitations of space and movement while traveling.*
- *When flying with infants, keep several bottles of juice or milk*

handy for ascending and descending. (Swallowing minimizes the possibility of earaches or other discomforts.)

The success of a trip depends most of all on your own attitude and state of mind. If you can relax, be flexible, understand an infant's restlessness and tiredness, give him a lot of attention (singing songs, telling stories, and encouraging him to observe the changing scenery when possible), the trip can be enjoyable for everyone.

Early December (20½ Months)

We are having spaghetti for dinner tonight, a family favorite. Mirabai is very hungry and walking underfoot while I am preparing it, saying over and over again, "Bibai have 'getti." It is driving me slightly mad. I suppose repetition is part of this stage of development, but I hope she grows out of it soon. My sons untactfully remind me that I do the same thing, but the comparison is unfair. At least I let hours and even days pass between my reiterations.

I knew that neither Mirabai nor I would be able to wait for dinner, so I boiled a handful of spinach pastina. This dish took only five minutes to cook and looked lovely served with tomato sauce. Mirabai hesitated to eat it because it wasn't the spaghetti she had expected, but hunger ruled and she finished it as well as a small lettuce and tomato salad.

Pasta belongs to one of the four basic food groups we need each day, the bread-cereal group that provides starch, bulk, and proteins, vitamins, and minerals. Pasta supplies us with carbohydrates. Made predominantly from wheat, it may contain other ingredients, such as soy, eggs, and spinach. Pasta plays an important role in the Italian diet, and there are many dozens of different shapes and types. All supermarkets carry a variety of macaroni products, but for the best selection it is worthwhile finding an Italian market.

Most children love pasta and there are limitless ways to serve it, from a simple spaghetti with olive oil and garlic to salad primavera. For infants and toddlers there is a special pastina (tiny dough) that can be prepared as a breakfast cereal with milk and raisins or fruit.

It can also be mixed with formula, milk, or butter, served as a side dish, added to soups, or mixed with vegetables. There are several other small pastas that children love, including stelline *(little stars),* alphabet, acini di pepe *(peppercorns),* orzo *(rice-shaped),* semi di mellone *(apple or melon seeds),* tubettini *(small hollow tubes),* ditalini *(larger hollow tubes), and* rotelle *(small wheels). They all mix well with squash, lentils, beans, fresh peas, chick-peas, broccoli, or spinach as well as with traditional tomato or meat sauces and fish, cheese, and meat dishes.*

If your child rejects a specific vegetable, he may accept it if mixed with pasta. With some experimentation, you will find unlimited combinations of this versatile food from which your child will choose his own favorites.

Mid-December (21 Months)

Christmas is rapidly approaching and today Mirabai tried her hand at making Christmas cookies for the first time with some help from Mommy, William, and her little friend Daniel. I prepared the mixture for *sirup snipper* (ginger snaps), a traditional Norwegian Christmas cookie, and let the children make the designs either freehand or with cookie cutters. William made a spectacular space shuttle, Daniel produced a tray of Santas, angels, stars, and trees, plus E.T., and Mirabai had a wonderful time pounding a piece of dough into a grayish rubbery substance until William taught her how to cut out a Santa Claus. After our creations had been in the oven for a few minutes, the house was filled with the wonderful aromas that remind me of past holidays.

Mirabai barely touched her dinner, having eaten too many cookies, not to mention a lot of raw dough. But for once I didn't worry, as she was having such a good time. Later we lit the fire and made popcorn, some of which we ate. The rest we threaded along with cranberries to trim the tree. Robert and his girlfriend made little paper baskets to hang on the tree that were filled with nuts, raisins, licorice, and chocolate. We placed them up high and told Mirabai that the chocolate was for Santa. Bob got into the spirit of things with a rousing and

somewhat inaccurate version of "Jingle Bells," so I started to
play some Christmas songs on the piano. Mirabai crawled up
beside me on the piano stool, and with her help Bob and I
sang a duet: the first time in our twenty-year marriage that
we have ever done such a thing.

Mirabai was too tired to help with the finishing touches on
the Christmas tree, and after one more song was quite willing
to be put to bed. As I tucked her in, she gave me a beautiful
smile and said, "I like cookies, Mama."

*Most Americans prize their cultural backgrounds, especially the
traditions and foods associated with them. As certain ethnic foods
may be difficult to obtain and their preparation very time-consuming,
many such dishes are prepared only on special holidays. At these
times I feel nutrition can take a backseat. Throughout the human life
cycle, food and eating serve not only to meet nutritional requirements
but are also important for personal psychosocial development. Conversation, warmth, and a happy atmosphere are as important as the
food served.*

Early January (21½ Months)

For Mirabai's lunch today I wanted to try something different, so I thought we would have fish. Growing up in Norway,
where wonderful fish was served almost daily, has made me
so particular about quality and freshness that I seldom buy it
here. However, it is not fair to deprive my family of this versatile and nutritious food they all love. So today I prepared
some fillets of sole and fresh spinach for our lunch. I steamed
the sole, washed the spinach and boiled it for five minutes in
the water clinging to the leaves, and cooked a few carrots.
Everything was ready in a few minutes, and I served it unsea-
soned with a dot of unsalted butter. Mirabai finished it all
with apparent pleasure, and then had a baked apple with raisins and milk for dessert.

*As our society becomes more calorie and nutrition conscious, fish
is becoming a frequent part of the diet. Fish is low in calories, and*

it is an excellent source of easily digested, high-quality protein, containing more polyunsaturated than saturated fats. The vitamin content varies with the species, but fish generally is a good source of riboflavin, niacin, and vitamin B_{12}. The fattier types of fish also supply the fat-soluble vitamin D. Fish contains significant amounts of phosphorus, potassium, magnesium, and iron, and is low in sodium. (Even saltwater fish are not high in sodium.) Because fish contains little connective tissue it is easy to digest and suitable for most diets.

Although fish is an excellent food source, many cooks resist preparing it, perhaps because they lack knowledge on how to cook it. Fish, when properly cooked, becomes opaque and flakes easily with a fork. Overcooking makes the flesh dry and tough. A good rule of thumb for judging if fish is perfectly cooked has been developed by the Canadian Department of Fisheries: Measure the fish at its thickest point. Allow ten minutes' cooking time for each inch of thickness for fresh fish, twenty minutes per inch for frozen fish. Fish may be cooked without thawing, except for layered fillets, which need to be partially thawed so that they can be separated. If fish is cooked in oil or a sauce, allow an extra five minutes per inch. Since there are many variables, always test fish to ensure that it is cooked through.

Another deterrent for many people is dealing with the skin and bones. Small bones are especially dangerous for young children. In Norway there was a method of preparing fish that was very popular when I was a child. It contained no skin or bones. Fish fillets were ground and made into a thick purée from which fish pudding, fish balls, or fish cakes could be made. I remember that my parents would need to set aside a whole day to prepare such dishes. Today, using a food processor, and with fish already skinned and boned, preparation would take little more than half an hour. For adults this may not be the most appealing way to eat fish, as it is somewhat bland, but toddlers and children love it.

I was looking through an old Norwegian cookbook recently and found some of the following recipes listed in the index: Fish cotelettes, Fish pâté, Fish filets Béarnaise, Fish fricassee, Fish au gratin, Fish fried à la Mignon, Fish ragu, Fish roulettes, Fish Wienerschnitzel. You can see that in Scandinavia fish is prepared in many ways we usually think of as reserved for meat. This does show that there is a large variety of ways in which fish can be served. If you are willing to experiment and are open to new flavors and textures, nutrition and mealtimes can both gain new dimensions.

Mid-February (23 Months)

It has been raining almost daily for months now, quite a phenomenon for Southern California, and we have been using the fireplace frequently. The sounds of wood crackling and rain against the windows and the coziness of the living room are all invitations for hot chocolate, popcorn, and a good book in front of the fire. This evening I made Bob cocoa with artificial sweetener, hot chocolate for the boys, and Mirabai and I had carob milk. Everyone had his own bowl of popcorn.

Mirabai loves these special evenings. Tonight we all took turns reading a story from her little library, which is geared toward two-year-olds. When the boys were very young we did the same thing, and I remember that fairy tales from other lands became great favorites. As they grew older the books matured with them. I later realized that reading aloud to the boys from a very early age helped lay the foundations for their love of reading. If I was not able to finish a story for two or three days, they became impatient to know the ending. Once they had learned to read, they would painstakingly work their way through the pages and soon were very proficient readers. But on rainy days we would still read aloud in front of the fire while sipping hot chocolate and eating popcorn.

Carob is a good substitute for chocolate. If you start your child on it, he will enjoy the flavor and eventually choose it over cocoa or chocolate. Carob powder is made from the dried pods of the carob tree, and its texture is similar to that of cocoa, although different in taste and nutritional value. It is higher in natural sugars, crude fiber, and iron, and lower in calories, crude fat, and sodium. Carob can be used as a substitute for cocoa or chocolate, and in recipes calling for cocoa the cocoa can be replaced by an equivalent amount of carob. When substituting chocolate in cooking, use 3 tablespoonsful of carob powder plus 1 tablespoonful of water for each square of chocolate. Carob blends well with other flavors and is especially good with orange, lemon, vanilla, and almond.

Not everyone has a fireplace, but family evenings with a warm atmosphere can be created in any household. Such occasions will lin-

ger in the memory for a lifetime. If pastimes, like games, reading, singing, crafts, or discussions, are part of the evening, a love for such activities will be fostered in your child in later years. This is worth keeping in mind especially when encouraging enthusiastic and proficient readers.

Mid-March (2 Years Old)

It is Mirabai's birthday and we are having a big party. I am not only celebrating her birthday but also the birth of this book, since we just signed the contract with our publisher. (Without Mirabai, however, there would have been no book!) We are inviting all the friends who have given encouragement, inspiration, or positive critiques. I have prepared a vegetarian lasagna, a huge green salad, and a Norwegian birthday cake. Jeannie is fixing some kind of exotic Thai chicken dish and a *tabbouleh* salad, Jana has made fruit salad, and Benita is bringing handmade chocolate baskets filled with chocolate-dipped strawberries and white-chocolate baskets full of delicious truffles and chocolates. To round out the buffet, we have lots of French bread and butter, wine, and soft drinks for the children.

I keep thinking that this is not a children's party, although there will be six of them present. It is basically my celebration of Mirabai's birth and the two years of love and happiness she has given us.

The Limoges china and crystal used for special occasions are dusted off and the silver has been shined. We have camellias, Easter lilies, and irises from the garden in every room in the house, and a fire is going in the living room because it is pouring rain outside. Two wonderful friends, Fay and Barbara, arrived early this morning and, with a speed, efficiency, and harmony rarely seen, cleaned, washed, polished, set the table, and decorated the house, leaving me time to prepare the food.

Mirabai knows something very special is happening today, her second birthday, and I am worried that she will be too excited to nap. But it is as if she knows she needs to sleep in order to be up this evening and goes willingly to bed, taking a three-hour nap. By the time she wakes up, Daddy is home. He gives her a bath, washes her hair, and dresses her in the prettiest dress she owns.

By the time the first guests arrive everything is ready, including me. This is a first! For once I don't have to greet my guests shoeless or with my hair uncombed. Mirabai opens her presents as each person arrives. In this way, it will not be too overwhelming for her and she can appreciate each gift and the person it is from. She is delighted when the children arrive, especially little Robert, who is three and a favorite friend. They wander off into Mirabai's room to play with her toys. All the children are well behaved but still having a good time. William and Daniel have disappeared. They are turning a cardboard box and bits of electrical gadgetry into a car and appear only to have their plates and glasses refilled. Little Christopher, also two, appears *au naturel*, informing his mother that his diaper was wet so he took it off. The adults, who range from eighteen to eighty-plus, are tucking into the food, socializing, and enjoying themselves.

Although Jeannie has done her utmost to talk me out of giving my little speech, I insist; so everyone's glass gets filled and the room becomes quiet. I give thanks and propose toasts for all the inspiration, ideas, and help given to *The Baby Cookbook*, and Mirabai gets her "Happy Birthday" song with much clapping, kissing, and hugs, and she is loving every minute of it. She is also very tired. Although the party is not over, she doesn't resist being put to bed. Soon other parents with children leave, and by the time the embers from the fire die down, the last guest says good-bye. It is the end of a busy, wonderful day. It is also the end of Mirabai's first two years in this world. We are entering into a new era, The Terrible Twos! But the memories of the last two years give me nothing but joy.

Part 2

FAMILY RECIPES AND SPECIAL CHILDREN'S RECIPES

Recipes

Notes on the Recipes

MOST of the recipes that follow, you would expect to find in an adult cookbook, not in *The Baby Cookbook*. So why are they included here? There are two reasons.

First, by the time your baby is twelve months old, he can share family meals. It is then important that he be exposed to as wide a variety of healthy foods as possible. Through a varied diet, he will acquire the taste for many foods from each of the four food groups, which should give him total nutrition. Your child's pleasure in eating will also be expanded and you will be discouraging him from becoming a finicky eater.

Second, *The Baby Cookbook* family recipes have been designed to be low in sodium (salt); they contain almost no sugar or refined sweeteners, emphasize high-quality foods and healthy methods of preparation, and are generally geared toward encouraging good eating habits. (Some adults may wish to add more salt and seasonings to suit their own tastes. This should be done only *after* your child's portion has been set aside for him. Your baby does not have your taste buds and does not need added salt.)

Recipes designed especially for very young children are mingled with family recipes that they can share when they are a little older, because, after all, your baby is certainly a member of the family, and all the family cooking takes place in one kitchen.

However, so that you can locate the special recipes for babies, the "serving" line at the bottom of those recipes is printed in **bold-face type** (such as **1 child serving**), and the titles of the recipes are identified in the same way in the Recipe Index. If you are alone with your baby at lunch or supper, there are some recipes that *you* can share with him: The serving line reads **1 adult and 1 child serving.** Or you can use such a recipe to make child portions for several meals.

Servings in the adult recipes vary in number so that the recipes can be used for two, four, six, or more people, or can be divided into two or more meals—one for now, the remainder for tomorrow's lunch or the freezer (which will help working mothers). A few recipes are for parties, to serve lots of people, and your child may have his share of those, too. All servings shown for adults are large enough to include some for your child, as he will need no more than one or two tablespoonful of each food from the meal.

You will discover that cooking well for the whole family is a great time-saver as your baby becomes a toddler and shares in family meals instead of having his food cooked for him separately.

PREPARATION OF BASIC FOODS

Dried Beans

There are two methods of preparing dried beans: One is to cook them without soaking; the other is to soak them overnight, which will considerably shorten the cooking time. In fact, unsoaked beans take twice as long to cook and twice as much water to prepare; there is also a greater risk of their burning or cooking dry, as they absorb the water more rapidly than presoaked beans.

A faster method than soaking beans overnight is to boil them in water for 2 minutes and then allow to stand for 1 hour.

There is some dispute over whether the water used for soaking should be saved, as it may contain valuable nutrients. According to the California Dry Bean Advisory Board, the nutrient loss is minimal when you discard the water. In addition to getting rid of impurities such as dirt or stones, soaking reduces flatus-causing factors, which are washed out in the soaking water (thus improving the digestibility of beans). The protein value of the beans is not affected, so it would seem advisable to discard the water.

Adding 1 tablespoonful of oil for each cup of beans during presoaking will reduce foaming that occurs when the beans are boiling.

One cup of dried beans will make about 3 cups of cooked beans.

2¼ cups dry beans (1 lb.),   OR FOR SMALLER QUANTITY
  presoaked   1 cup dry beans, presoaked
7 cups water   4 cups water

METHOD ONE

Bring water to a boil in a heavy kettle. Beans should first be sorted carefully and washed in cold water and drained. Add beans to boiling water, return to a boil, and cook over high heat for 2 minutes. Remove from heat and let stand for at least 1 hour. Drain, rinse, replace water, and bring to a boil again. Reduce heat and simmer, covered, until tender (from 1 to 2 hours, depending on the type of bean). Drain.

METHOD TWO

Add presoaked beans to rapidly boiling water. Return to boil, reduce heat, cover, and simmer until tender. Drain.

In both methods check during cooking to ensure that beans do not burn or dry out. If too much water evaporates, add more as necessary.

o o o

Lentils

Lentils do not require soaking before cooking. Using 1 cup of lentils to 3 cups of water, these legumes can be prepared in the same way as dried beans (Method Two). Cooking time will be between 40 and 60 minutes.

One cup of uncooked lentils will make about 2 cups of cooked lentils.

o o o

Tomatoes
(How to Blanch and Peel)

Add a whole tomato to a small pan of boiling water. Remove from heat. Let stand for 1 minute. Remove with a slotted spoon, cool a little, then remove skin with a sharp paring knife.

o o o

Stewed Fruit

Clean, pit, and peel fruit. Use ripe sweet fruits such as apples, peaches, plums, etc. Place fruit with enough water to cover in a small saucepan. Gently bring to a boil, reduce heat and simmer until tender, around 10 to 15 minutes. Drain off liquid, or use when puréeing the fruit.

If the fruit is too sharp or acidic for your baby, add a little mashed banana or papaya.

Dried fruits may be stewed. It is not necessary, or easy, to peel them. Use the same method as for fresh fruits, although cooking times may vary a little.

○ ○ ○

Homemade Yogurt

2 cups whole milk
¼ cup dry nonfat milk
Bulgarian yogurt starter (obtainable in freeze-dried packet
    from health-food stores)

Check directions on yogurt starter packet for how much to use for 2 cups milk. Mix whole and nonfat milks together in a saucepan and heat almost to boiling point. Remove from heat and cool to 90°–100° (test with food thermometer). Add yogurt starter and stir until completely dissolved. Pour mixture into a meticulously clean container, cover with lid, and keep warm until yogurt is set. (I keep mine warm on top of the stove with a sweater wrapped around it.) After 6 to 8 hours, when yogurt is firm, place in refrigerator and let stand overnight.

For the next batch of yogurt, use a tablespoonful from this recipe as a starter.

MAKES ABOUT 2 CUPS

o o o

Paneer
(Homemade Cottage Cheese)

½ gallon whole or low-fat milk
Juice of 2 lemons

Bring milk to a foaming boil over medium heat and add the lemon juice. Stir together briefly and allow milk to boil for a few more seconds until it curdles. Remove pan from heat and let stand until curds and whey separate (2 to 3 minutes). Using a clean cheesecloth or sieve, strain off liquid and refrigerate cheese in a covered container until needed.

Be sure to save whey liquid to use in soups or drinks. It is highly nutritious.

MAKES ½ CUP

VEGETABLES

Baked Acorn Squash

1 acorn (or butternut) squash
2 tbsp. butter or margarine

Scrub squash, halve, and scoop out seeds. Put 1 tablespoon butter or margarine in each half and place in an ovenproof dish containing 1 inch of water. Cover with foil and bake in preheated 350° oven for about 1 hour, or until tender. Remove flesh from shells and mash, adding more butter, or milk, if needed.

Salt and pepper may be added for adults, if desired.

SERVES 2

○ ○ ○

Asparagus with Parmesan Cheese

1 bunch fresh asparagus, washed and trimmed
2 tbsp. olive oil
⅓ cup freshly grated Parmesan cheese

Stand asparagus upright in a tall saucepan half filled with boiling water, and cook until semisoft but the bottoms of the spears are still firm when tested with a knife. Drain well and arrange in a baking dish. Baste with the olive oil and sprinkle with the Parmesan cheese. Bake in preheated 400° oven for about 10 minutes, or until cheese browns.

SERVES 4

○ ○ ○

Avocado and Papaya Salad

1 ripe avocado   ½ ripe papaya

DRESSING

¼ cup lime juice   ⅛ tsp. pepper
¼ tsp. salt   ¼ cup olive oil

Peel and seed avocado and papaya and slice into a bowl. Mix together lime juice, salt, and pepper, and stir in olive oil until blended. Use half of dressing to cover salad (reserving remainder in refrigerator for another use).
    Dressing may be omitted for young children, if preferred.

SERVES 2

o o o

Stuffed Bell Peppers

4 large bell peppers,
  washed, tops removed,
  and seeded
3 tbsp. butter or margarine
1 small onion, peeled and
  chopped
12 mushrooms, washed and
  sliced
1 cup cooked rice

¼ cup seedless raisins
½ cup bread crumbs
1½ cups canned tomatoes,
  crushed
4 tbsp. grated Cheddar
  cheese
1 cup tomato sauce
  (optional; see page 283)

Set peppers in a pan of boiling water for 1 minute. Remove
and place in ovenproof baking dish. Melt butter or margarine
in a skillet and sauté onion and mushrooms until tender. Add
rice, raisins, bread crumbs, and tomatoes and mix well, but
do not cook. With a spoon narrow enough to fit inside the
peppers, fill each pepper to the top with mixture. Add ¼ cup
water to baking dish and cook peppers in preheated 350° oven
for 30 minutes. Eight minutes before peppers are done, sprinkle tops with grated cheese. Serve with tomato sauce, if desired.

SERVES 4

o o o

Broccoli Indian Style

½ lb. broccoli, washed and
  cut up
1 tbsp. safflower or peanut
  oil
1 tsp. mustard seeds

1 onion, peeled and
  chopped
1 tsp. turmeric

½ tsp. coriander

1 tsp. *garam masala* (from Far Eastern grocery store; or see page 153)

1 tbsp. lemon juice

2 tbsp. plain yogurt

1 tbsp. shredded coconut

¼ cup water

2 tomatoes, peeled and chopped (optional)

Steam broccoli for 5 minutes (it should still be quite firm). In pan heat oil and add mustard seeds. Stir while they pop, then reduce heat to medium, add onion, and sauté until tender. Add turmeric, coriander, *garam masala*, lemon juice, yogurt, coconut, and water (also tomatoes, if desired). Mix well, bring to a boil, and add broccoli. Reduce heat and let simmer for 5 minutes, or until flavors have blended and broccoli is tender.

SERVES 2

○ ○ ○

Garam Masala
(Indian Seasoning)

Seeds from 2 cardamom pods

30 whole peppercorns

1 tsp. whole cloves

2 tsp. whole cumin seeds (optional)

2-inch piece cinnamon stick

Grind all ingredients as finely as possible, using either a mortar and pestle or a nut grinder. Store in an airtight container, as this supply will last some time.

o o o

Brussels Sprouts and Carrots in Lemon Butter

½ lb. Brussels sprouts,
  trimmed and halved
½ lb. carrots, scrubbed and
  halved lengthwise and
  crosswise

4 tbsp. butter or margarine
1 small clove garlic, minced
Juice and grated peel of ¼
  lemon

Steam Brussels sprouts and carrots for 10 minutes. Drain and arrange in a heated serving dish. Melt butter or margarine with garlic, add lemon juice and peel, and pour over vegetables. (Save stock from vegetables for other recipes.)

SERVES 4

o o o

Carrot Apple Purée

1 carrot, scrubbed and sliced
1 apple, peeled, cored, and
  sliced
2 tbsp. milk
½ tsp. butter or margarine

Steam carrot and apple slices until tender. Purée or mash with milk and butter or margarine

2 OR 3 CHILD SERVINGS

○ ○ ○

Carrots and Beets with Apple

2 medium-size carrots,
  scrubbed and thinly sliced
2 small cooked beets, diced

½ apple, cored, washed,
  and diced
⅓ cup apple juice
1 tbsp. finely chopped
  parsley

Simmer carrots, beets, and apple in apple juice until tender, about 10 minutes. Purée or mash to desired consistency and top with parsley.

1 ADULT AND 1 CHILD SERVING

○ ○ ○

Carrot Raita

8 oz. plain yogurt (see page
  149 for homemade)
½ carrot, scrubbed and
  finely grated

1 tbsp. raisins, soaked in
  water for 30 minutes
Dash ground cardamom

Whip yogurt lightly in a bowl. Add carrot, soaked and drained raisins, and a tiny dash of cardamom, and mix well. Chill before serving.

1 ADULT AND 1 CHILD SERVING

○ ○ ○

Cauliflower with Avocado-Tahini Dressing

1 large head cauliflower,
   green leaves removed,
   washed and left whole
1 bay leaf

1 ripe avocado, peeled and
   pitted
1 cup tahini dressing (see
   page 285)

Place cauliflower in a steamer, add bay leaf, and steam until tender but still firm. Remove bay leaf and place cauliflower in a preheated dish. Mash avocado and mix with tahini dressing until smooth. Pour over cauliflower and serve immediately.

SERVES 6

○ ○ ○

Pineapple Coleslaw

½ cup plain yogurt
¼ cup light mayonnaise
2 cups shredded cabbage

½ cup grated carrot
½ cup fresh or canned
   crushed pineapple,
   drained

Mix yogurt with mayonnaise in a large bowl. Combine cabbage, carrots, and pineapple, and stir into yogurt-mayonnaise mixture, blending well. Chill.

SERVES 6

○ ○ ○

Cucumber Salad

1 large cucumber, peeled
  and thinly sliced
½ tsp. salt for preparation of
  cucumber

1 cup plain yogurt
1 tsp. dill
Dash white pepper

Put cucumber in a bowl, sprinkle with salt, and let stand for 1 hour. Drain off any accumulated liquid, add yogurt, dill, and pepper, and blend well. May be chilled before serving.

SERVES 3 TO 4

○ ○ ○

Eggplant Parmesan

2 medium-size eggplant,
  unpeeled
Salt for preparation of
  eggplant
Olive oil

2 cups tomato sauce (see
  page 283)
1 lb. mozzarella cheese,
  thinly sliced
¼ lb. Parmesan cheese,
  grated

Wash eggplant and cut into slices ¾ inch thick. Lay slices on paper towels, sprinkle with salt, and cover with more towels. Weight down with heavy pots, etc., and let stand for 1 to 2 hours. Then brush liberally with olive oil and put under pre-heated broiler to brown, turning once.

Cover bottom of a lasagna pan, or other large ovenproof dish, with thin layer of tomato sauce, cover this with layer of eggplant slices, add more sauce and a layer of mozzarella, and sprinkle with Parmesan cheese. Repeat the layers one more time, and cover dish with foil. Bake in preheated 350° oven for 30 minutes, or until sauce bubbles and cheese is melted. Serve immediately.

SERVES 6

o o o

Sweet and Savory Eggplant

½ cucumber, peeled and
　halved lengthwise
¼ cup olive or corn oil
1 clove garlic, finely
　chopped
1 medium-size eggplant,
　unpeeled, washed, and
　cubed

1 bell pepper, washed,
　seeded, and thinly sliced
1 tsp. tarragon
2 tomatoes, peeled and
　chopped
⅓ cup fresh or canned
　crushed pineapple
2 tbsp. chopped parsley

Cut cucumber into ½-inch slices. Heat oil in a large skillet, add garlic, eggplant, pepper, cucumber, and tarragon, mix well, and simmer over low flame until all ingredients are tender. Add chopped tomatoes and pineapple, mix well, and heat through. Sprinkle with parsley and serve with rice.

SERVES 2

o o o

Green Beans with Walnuts

2 tbsp. olive oil
1 clove garlic, mashed
¼ cup ground walnuts
1 cup French-style green
　beans, cooked

Heat oil in a frying pan, add mashed garlic, ground walnuts, and green beans. Mix gently and toss beans until well blended and heated through.

SERVES 2

o o o

Indian Vegetables with Rice

4 tbsp. safflower oil
1 tsp. mustard seeds
1 large clove garlic, crushed
1 medium-size onion,
  peeled and sliced thin
3 potatoes, peeled and
  chopped
5 carrots, scraped and
  chopped
½ head each cabbage and
  cauliflower, washed and
  chopped
1 small bunch broccoli,
  washed and cut into
  florets

1 cup tomato sauce, fresh
  (see page 283) or canned
1 tsp. sesame salt
1-inch piece fresh ginger,
  grated, or ½ tsp. ground
  ginger
½ tsp. chili powder
2 tomatoes, peeled (if
  desired) and chopped
Parsley, chopped, for
  garnish

Heat oil in a large heavy pan, add mustard seeds, and cook until they pop. Add garlic and onion, and cook until glazed. Add potatoes and sauté gently for 5 minutes. Add carrots, cabbage, cauliflower, and broccoli to pan, plus tomato sauce, sesame salt, ginger, and chili powder. Simmer until vegetables are tender, adding stock or water as needed. Add chopped tomatoes at the last minute. Serve over rice on a heated platter, and sprinkle with chopped parsley.

SERVES 4 TO 6

o o o

Stuffed Mushrooms

6 large mushrooms,   ½ cup grated Cheddar
  washed, stems removed   cheese
1 tbsp. butter or margarine   3 tsp. bread crumbs
                            1 tbsp. chopped parsley

Cover mushroom caps with boiling water for 2 minutes,
drain, and dry. Place mushrooms in a buttered pie dish, put
a pat of butter or margarine inside each cap, and pop under
preheated broiler until almost tender. Add a generous helping
of grated cheese to each cap, sprinkle with bread crumbs, and
return to broiler until cheese is melted and crisp. Garnish with
parsley and serve immediately.

SERVES 2 TO 3

o o o

Green Peas with Pineapple

½ cup green peas, fresh or frozen
1 tbsp. finely chopped fresh or canned pineapple
1 small ripe tomato, peeled and finely chopped

In a small saucepan put peas, pineapple, and tomato, including juices from pineapple and tomato. Cook over low heat
until tender, stirring occasionally. Purée or mash to desired
consistency.

2 OR 3 CHILD SERVINGS

o o o

Heavenly Potato

1 large potato, peeled
3 tbsp. cream, warmed (not boiled)
2 tbsp. grated Cheddar cheese
1 tbsp. butter or margarine, melted

Boil potato until soft and mash with cream. Put into a small heat-proof dish, top with grated cheese, and cover with the melted butter or margarine. Pop under preheated broiler until cheese is melted and serve.

1 ADULT AND 1 CHILD SERVING

o o o

Swedish Potato Pancakes

1 medium-size potato,
   peeled and grated
1 egg, beaten
2 tsp. flour
1 tbsp. vegetable oil

Squeeze all moisture from grated potato. Add beaten egg and flour to potato and mix well. Heat oil in a skillet, add potato mixture by tablespoonsful, and fry pancakes until brown. Turn and continue to cook until brown on the other side. Serve with applesauce or mashed banana.

MAKES 6 SMALL PANCAKES

o o o

Mashed Rutabaga and Carrots

1 small rutabaga, peeled
   and cubed
2 carrots, scrubbed and
   sliced
1 tbsp. butter or margarine
Dash white pepper
   (optional)

Steam rutabaga and carrots until tender. Mash vegetables
with butter or margarine and pepper to desired consistency
(or purée in a blender or food processor for younger baby).

1 ADULT AND 1 CHILD SERVING

o o o

Semolina Primavera

1 large onion, chopped
1 clove garlic, minced
1 tbsp. butter or margarine,
   or 2 tbsp. peanut or
   olive oil
1½ cups homemade chicken
   stock (see page 280)
1 red or green sweet pepper,
   diced

1 tbsp. chopped fresh basil
   or oregano (or 1 tsp.
   dried)
1 zucchini, diced
1 large or 2 small ripe
   tomatoes, peeled and
   chopped
1 cup semolina (couscous)
2 tbsp. minced fresh parsley
3 tbsp. grated Parmesan
   cheese

In a large pot sauté onion and garlic in butter, margarine, or
oil until tender. Add chicken stock, pepper, and basil or oreg-

ano, cover, and simmer for 5 minutes. Then add zucchini and simmer for 3 minutes more, stirring occasionally. Add tomatoes and semolina and stir for 1 minute or until semolina is thoroughly moistened. Cover tightly and remove from heat. Let stand for 5 minutes, then fluff lightly with a fork. Sprinkle with parsley and Parmesan cheese before serving.

SERVES 6

o o o

Spinach and Potato Casserole

4 medium-size potatoes,
  peeled and sliced
4 eggs, beaten
¼ lb. (1 stick) butter or
  margarine, melted

2 cups grated Cheddar or
  Swiss cheese
Two 10-oz. packages frozen
  chopped spinach, cooked
  and drained

In an oiled ovenproof dish make a layer of half the potato slices. Combine the eggs, melted butter or margarine, and grated cheese, and pour half the mixture over potatoes. Follow with a layer of all the spinach, making sure it is well drained. Add another layer of potatoes and cover with the rest of the egg, butter, and cheese mixture. Cover and bake in preheated 350° oven for 1¼ hours.

SERVES 4 TO 6

o o o

Spinach Yogurt Bake

1 lb. fresh spinach, washed,
　or 10-oz. package frozen
　chopped spinach
2 tbsp. butter or margarine

1 small onion, peeled and
　chopped
2 tbsp. flour
1 cup plain yogurt
1 cup grated jack cheese

Cook fresh spinach in covered pot, using only water left on
leaves, for 3 minutes, stirring occasionally. (Cook frozen spinach according to package directions.) Drain well. Heat butter
or margarine in a skillet and sauté onion in it until soft. Add
flour and stir over medium heat for 1 minute. Gradually
whisk in yogurt and mix well, followed by spinach, which
should be stirred to coat with yogurt and onion, and heat
through. Remove from heat and blend in grated cheese until
melted. Pour mixture into greased 8×4-inch loaf pan and
bake in preheated 350° oven for 20 minutes.

SERVES 2

o o o

Cheesy Baked Squash

1 summer squash
1 small zucchini
1 yellow crookneck squash
5 mushrooms
½ onion, peeled
1 red pepper, seeded

¼ cup olive oil
1 clove garlic, peeled and
　mashed
¼ tsp. each oregano and
　basil
½ cup grated jack cheese
½ cup grated Parmesan
　cheese

Wash and slice all vegetables and steam together until tender. Meanwhile, combine olive oil, garlic, oregano, and basil. Transfer vegetables to an ovenproof casserole and cover with olive oil mixture and then with the grated cheeses. Cover and bake in preheated 350° oven for 20 minutes. Remove cover and bake for another 10 minutes.

SERVES 4

o o o

Squash with Green Beans

1 young acorn squash,
   halved and seeded
4 tbsp. butter or margarine
½ cup green beans, washed
   and trimmed

2 tbsp. grated Parmesan
   cheese
1 tsp. finely chopped
   parsley

Dot each squash half with 1 tablespoon butter or margarine and bake in preheated 375° oven for 20 minutes, or until tender. Meanwhile, steam green beans until tender, then cut into ½-inch pieces; toss with remaining 2 tablespoons butter or margarine. Fill both halves of squash with beans, top with Parmesan cheese, and sprinkle with parsley.

SERVES 2

o o o

Summer Salad

½ cup plain yogurt
½ cup light mayonnaise
½ cup diced steamed green
  beans
½ cup diced cooked potato
½ cup diced steamed carrot

½ cup diced cooked beet
½ cup cucumber, peeled and
  diced
½ cup diced fresh or canned
  pineapple
4 hard-boiled eggs, diced

In a large bowl blend yogurt and mayonnaise well, then add all other ingredients. Mix together gently until coated and refrigerate until ready to serve.

SERVES 6

o o o

Sweet Potato and Apple Purée

1 small sweet potato or yam,
  peeled and sliced
½ apple, peeled, cored, and
  sliced
½ tsp. butter or margarine
2 tbsp. milk

Steam sweet potato and apple slices until tender. Purée or mash to desired consistency with butter or margarine and milk.

2 OR 3 CHILD SERVINGS

o o o

Sweet Potato Scramble

3 tbsp. butter or margarine   1 egg, beaten
1 sweet potato (or yam),   1 tbsp. shredded jack cheese
   cooked and sliced   ½ tsp. chopped parsley

Melt 2 tablespoons butter or margarine in a skillet and sauté
sweet potato slices in it until golden brown. In a small pan
melt remaining butter or margarine and scramble egg over
low heat, adding jack cheese and stirring until cheese is
melted. Put sweet potato slices on a warm plate, cover with
egg mixture, sprinkle with parsley, and serve immediately.

1 ADULT AND 1 CHILD SERVING

o o o

Broiled Tomato

1 firm medium-size tomato   ¼ tsp. lemon juice (optional)
1 tbsp. chopped parsley   1 tsp. butter or margarine
1 tsp. bread crumbs (or
   grated Parmesan cheese)

Wash tomato and cut in half. Sprinkle with parsley, bread
crumbs, and lemon juice (if desired). Dot with butter or margarine and pop under preheated broiler for 5 minutes. Cut up
1 tomato half to serve to a child.

SERVES 2

o o o

Stuffed Tomato Treat

1 small firm tomato, washed   1 tbsp. shredded Swiss or
1 tbsp. butter or margarine   jack cheese
1 egg   ½ tsp. chopped parsley

Cut top off tomato, scoop out pulp and save, but discard hard
core and seeds. Melt butter or margarine in a small skillet and
scramble egg in it with tomato pulp. Fill tomato with mixture,
top with shredded cheese, and place in a small pan with water to cover bottom. Bake for 15 to 20 minutes in preheated
350° oven until tomato is soft and cheese is melted. Sprinkle
with parsley and serve.

1 CHILD SERVING

o o o

Tomato Eggplant Cups

¼ cup diced steamed   1 tsp. grated Parmesan
   eggplant   cheese
¼ cup cooked rice   1 tsp. finely chopped
2 firm medium-size   parsley
   tomatoes, washed   1 tsp. bread crumbs

Purée eggplant in a blender or food processor and mix with
cooked rice. Cut tops off tomatoes and scoop out cores and
pulp. Discard cores, add pulp to eggplant and rice, and spoon
mixture into tomato shells. Combine Parmesan cheese with
parsley and bread crumbs, and spoon on top of eggplant filling. Place in a greased ovenproof dish and bake in a pre-

heated 350° oven for 15 to 20 minutes, or until tomatoes are tender.

SERVES 2

○ ○ ○

Creamy Turnip

1 turnip, peeled and cut into   2 tbsp. milk
   small pieces   1 tbsp. butter or margarine
                                        ¼ tsp. grated lemon rind

Steam turnip until very soft. Mash well with all other ingredients, or purée to desired consistency. This method also works well with parsnips or rutabagas.

2 OR 3 CHILD SERVINGS

○ ○ ○

Vegetable Custard

2 egg yolks
¼ cup milk
¼ cup puréed vegetables (carrots, peas, sweet potato, etc.)

Beat egg yolks and mix with milk and puréed vegetables. Pour into 2 buttered custard cups and bake in preheated 350° oven until set.

2 CHILD SERVINGS

o o o

Vegetable Rice Casserole

1 small cauliflower, trimmed and cut into florets
2 medium-size carrots, scrubbed and sliced
1 stalk celery, washed and sliced

4 tbsp. peanut or vegetable oil
1 cup rice, rinsed
5 cups chicken or vegetable stock (see page 280 or page 281)
1 tbsp. chopped parsley

Sauté cauliflower, carrots, and celery in oil over low heat for 5 minutes, stirring to prevent sticking. Add rice and sauté for 2 more minutes. Grease a 2-quart ovenproof dish, add vegetables and rice, and pour stock over mixture. Cover and bake in preheated 375° oven for approximately 1 hour until rice and vegetables are tender. Sprinkle with parsley.

For children, mash or purée to desired consistency.

SERVES 4

o o o

Yam and Carrot Balls with Raisins

¼ cup raisins
½ cup orange juice
1 medium-size yam or sweet potato, peeled and sliced
2 medium-size carrots, scrubbed and sliced

¼ small onion, peeled and chopped
1 tbsp. olive oil
1 tsp. grated orange rind
½ tsp. grated lemon rind
Chopped parsley

Soak raisins in orange juice while steaming yam and carrots. Sauté onion in the oil until tender and drain. When yam and carrots are tender, mash with a little of the orange juice, drain the raisins, and add along with all other ingredients except parsley to mashed vegetables. The mixture should be firm enough to hold together. Using a tablespoon, make little balls and place in a well-greased ovenproof casserole. Bake in pre-heated 375° oven for 20 minutes. Sprinkle with parsley before serving.

1 ADULT AND 1 CHILD SERVING

o o o

Stuffed Zucchini with Apricot

1 large zucchini
2 tbsp. vegetable oil
½ onion, peeled and
   chopped
⅓ cup long-grained or
   basmati rice
1 medium-size tomato,
   peeled and chopped

1 cup vegetable or chicken
   stock (see page 281 or
   page 280)
⅓ cup diced cooked
   apricots, with juice
1 tsp. lemon juice

Halve the zucchini lengthwise and scrape out pulp (but save), leaving shell approximately ¾ inch thick. Boil shells in water to cover for 3 minutes and drain well. Heat oil in a large skillet and in it sauté onion and zucchini pulp until tender. Add rice, tomato, and broth, bring to a boil, cover, and cook for 15 minutes over low heat. Place half the apricots in an ovenproof dish with 4 tablespoons of their juice, add zucchini shells filled with the rice-zucchini mixture, and top with remainder of apricots. Sprinkle with lemon juice and bake in preheated 350° oven for 30 minutes, basting frequently with pan juices.
   Purée serving for infants in blender.

SERVES 2

○ ○ ○

Zucchini Mushroom Pie

12 mushrooms, washed and
   sliced
4 green onions, washed and
   sliced
1 tbsp. butter or margarine
4 zucchini, washed and
   grated

1 cup grated Cheddar or
   jack cheese
½ cup grated Parmesan
   cheese
½ cup wheat germ or bread
   crumbs
3 eggs, beaten
½ tsp. oregano

Sauté mushrooms and onions in butter or margarine until tender. Mix with zucchini, grated cheeses, wheat germ or bread
crumbs, eggs, and oregano. Press mixture into an 8- or 9-inch
greased pie dish and bake in preheated 350° oven for 35
minutes.

SERVES 6 TO 8

LEGUMES

Bean and Cheese Melt

1 cup mushrooms, washed
   and sliced
2 leeks, washed and sliced
2 tbsp. olive oil
1 tsp. oregano

2 cups cooked white beans
   (see page 146)
6 tomatoes, peeled and
   sliced
1 cup grated Swiss or jack
   cheese
Herb salt to taste (optional)

Sauté mushrooms and leeks in oil for 2 to 3 minutes until tender, and season with oregano. Put beans in an ovenproof dish, layer with sautéed vegetables and the tomatoes, and top with grated cheese and herb salt, if desired. Bake in preheated 325° oven for 15 minutes, or until cheese is bubbly.

SERVES 4

o o o

Cuban Black Beans

1½ cups cooked black beans
  (see page 146)
¼ cup bean cooking liquid
1 cup chopped seeded green
  peppers

1 cup chopped onions
2 tbsp. vegetable oil
1 bay leaf

Place beans in pan with their cooking liquid and heat gently. Sauté peppers and onions in vegetable oil for 5 minutes, or until tender. Drain any excess oil and add mixture to beans with the bay leaf. Continue to simmer for another 5 minutes, stirring occasionally. Remove bay leaf before serving.

SERVES 4

o o o

Peruvian Bean Purée

1 tbsp. chopped onion
1 tbsp. butter or margarine
¼ cup cooked lima beans
   (see page 146)
1 tbsp. chopped parsley

Sauté onion in butter or margarine until tender. Mash together with cooked lima beans, add parsley, and serve. May be puréed, if desired.

2 CHILD SERVINGS

o o o

Black-eyed Peas and Rice

16-oz. can black-eyed peas,
   or 1 cup dried black-eyed
   peas, freshly cooked (see
   page 146)
Water
½ cup rice

½ cup chopped onions
1 tsp. garlic salt
⅛ tsp. chili powder
1 cup shredded Cheddar
   cheese

Drain peas, reserving liquid. Add water to liquid until it measures 2½ cups. In a large skillet combine black-eyed peas, rice, onions, garlic salt, chili powder, and liquid. Stir, bring to a boil, cover, reduce heat, and simmer for 20 minutes. Remove from heat. Sprinkle with grated cheese, replace cover, and let stand until cheese is melted and all liquid has been absorbed, about 5 minutes.

SERVES 3 TO 4

○ ○ ○

Mild Vegetarian Chili with Beans

1 onion, peeled and
   chopped
2 tbsp. vegetable oil
3 tomatoes, peeled and
   chopped
½ cup tomato paste
½ tsp. basil
1 cup stock (from beans)

¼ tsp. oregano
¼ tsp. cumin
¼ tsp. garlic powder
1 cup pinto beans, cooked
   (see page 146)

Sauté onion in heated oil until golden, add all other ingredients except the beans, and heat through, stirring well to blend flavors. Combine ingredients with pinto beans and simmer for 20 minutes before serving.

SERVES 2

○ ○ ○

Garbanzo Bean Purée

½ cup cooked garbanzo
   beans (see page 146)
¼ cup tahini (sesame-seed
   paste)
¼ cup lemon juice

1 tbsp. olive oil
1 clove garlic, mashed
½ tsp. paprika
1 tbsp. minced parsley

Put all ingredients except paprika and parsley into a blender or food processor, and purée. Garnish with parsley and paprika. May be served as a dip with sliced carrots, celery, cauliflower, etc., or spread on crackers or pita bread.

MAKES ABOUT ¾ CUP

o o o

Lentil and Banana Mash

2 tbsp. cooked lentils (see page 148)
⅓ banana

Warm lentils, mash banana, and combine ingredients. Purée
for younger infants.

1 CHILD SERVING

o o o

Lentils Indian Style

1 cup lentils
1 tbsp. peanut or safflower
    oil
1 tsp. mustard seeds
1 clove garlic, crushed
¼ onion, peeled and
    chopped
¼ tsp. ground ginger

¼ tsp. *garam masala* (see
    page 153)
½ cup tomato purée
Grated Cheddar cheese
4 pita breads (see page 251)

Cook lentils (see page 148) until tender in a large pot. Drain.
Heat oil in a skillet and cook mustard seeds in it until they
pop. Add garlic and onion and sauté until golden. Add
ground ginger, *garam masala,* and tomato purée, stir well, and
cook for a few minutes. Add lentils and continue cooking for
another 15 minutes.

For older children and adults, put 1 to 2 tbsp. of grated
Cheddar cheese inside each pita bread and heat in oven until
cheese is melted. Serve immediately with lentils.

Serves 4

○ ○ ○

Lentil and Potato Stew

2 tbsp. lentils
½ potato, peeled and diced
1⅓ cups water
1 ripe tomato, peeled and
  chopped

¼ tsp. thyme
½ tsp. lemon juice
1 tsp. finely chopped
  parsley

Rinse lentils and put in a saucepan with potato and water. Bring to a boil, reduce heat, and simmer, covered, for 20 minutes. Add tomato and thyme, stir, and cook for another 5 to 10 minutes, still covered, over low heat. Add lemon juice, sprinkle with parsley, and serve.

2 OR 3 CHILD SERVINGS

○ ○ ○

Lentil Roast

2 tbsp. cooked lentils (see
  page 148)
1 small potato, cooked and
  mashed

¼ cup cooked peas
2 egg yolks, beaten
3 tbsp. grated Cheddar
  cheese

Grease an ovenproof dish, mix first four ingredients, and place in dish. Top with grated cheese and bake in preheated 325° oven for 30 minutes.

1 ADULT AND 1 CHILD SERVING

○ ○ ○

Lentils with Tomato and Celery

½ onion, peeled and
chopped
1 clove garlic, peeled and
mashed
2 stalks celery, washed and
finely chopped
1 tbsp. vegetable oil

¼ cup reserved lentil
cooking liquid
1 cup cooked lentils (see
page 148)
2 tomatoes, peeled and
chopped

Sauté onion, garlic, and celery in oil until tender and drain.
Add reserved liquid to lentils and heat through gently. Add
sautéed vegetables and tomatoes to lentils and simmer over
low heat for 5 minutes, stirring occasionally.

SERVES 4

○ ○ ○

Lima Beans

1 cup small dried lima
beans, washed
2½ cups water
1 tbsp. safflower oil
1 onion, peeled, finely
chopped, and sautéed

2 tomatoes, peeled,
chopped, and sautéed
1 tsp. minced parsley
Dash marjoram
1 tsp. vegetable salt
(optional)
Dash white pepper
(optional)

In a heavy pot place lima beans and water, bring to a boil,
and cook over high heat for 2 minutes. Remove from heat and
let stand for 1 hour. Then stir in oil, return to a boil, reduce
heat, and simmer for 45 minutes. In the last 5 minutes, add

onion, tomatoes, parsley, marjoram, and salt and pepper, if desired.

Serves 6

○ ○ ○

Frijoles I
(Refried Beans)

1 cup dried pinto beans, cooked (see page 146) and puréed	⅓ cup grated Cheddar cheese
1 small clove garlic, mashed	1 tsp. *tamari* or soy sauce
¼ cup grated onion	Pinch each basil and oregano

Mix all ingredients together and heat in a double boiler until cheese is melted and blended.

Serves 4

○ ○ ○

Frijoles II

¼ cup vegetable oil
1 cup dried pinto beans, cooked (see page 146)
½ cup grated Cheddar or jack cheese

Stir oil into cooked and heated beans and mash. Add grated cheese and continue to cook until cheese is completely melted.

Serves 4

o o o

Frijoles III

¼ cup corn oil
1 cup dried pinto beans,
    cooked (see page 146)
½ cup tomatoes, peeled and
    diced

¼ cup chopped onion
1 cup *queso fresco* cheese,
    crumbled

Heat oil in a skillet and add beans with a slotted spoon. Mash with a potato masher. Add water or broth, if necessary, to bring to desired consistency, stir in tomatoes and onion, and cook until onion is tender. Serve in individual bowls, topped with crumbled cheese.

SERVES 4

o o o

Soy Potato Burgers

1 cup dried soybeans,
    cooked (see page 146)
6 tbsp. chopped hazelnuts
2 raw potatoes, peeled and
    grated
1 onion, finely chopped

2 tbsp. milk
¼ tsp. salt
Vegetable oil for frying

Grind soybeans and hazelnuts in a blender or food processor, and combine with all other ingredients except oil. Form into small thin patties and sauté in a little oil over low heat until potatoes and onion are cooked through.

SERVES 4

o o o

Mini Tostadas

Package small tortillas
1 can vegetarian refried
  beans, or 1½ cups
  homemade (see pages
  179–180)

2 tomatoes, finely chopped
1 cup grated Cheddar
  cheese

Warm 6 tortillas in the oven according to directions on package. Gently heat the beans and spread a spoonful on each tortilla. Cover each with chopped tomato and sprinkle with grated cheese. Pop under preheated broiler for 2 or 3 minutes, or just until cheese is melted.

For older children and adults, shredded cooked chicken or cooked ground beef may be added, and the dish may be topped with olives and hot sauce.

MAKES 6 TOSTADAS

o o o

Small White Beans

1 onion, peeled and
  chopped
2 tbsp. vegetable oil
1 cup dried white beans,
  cooked (see page 146)
¼ cup reserved bean liquid

1 tomato, peeled and
  chopped
1 tbsp. chopped parsley

Sauté onion in oil until tender and drain. In a saucepan, combine ingredients and simmer for a few minutes to develop flavor, stirring to prevent sticking.

SERVES 4

TOFU

Tofu and Cauliflower

2 small cauliflowerets
2 oz. mashed tofu (approximately ¼ cup)
1 tbsp. shredded Cheddar cheese

Steam cauliflowerets for 10 minutes and mash together with tofu. Place mixture in a small heatproof dish, top with shredded cheese, and pop under preheated broiler until the cheese is melted.

1 CHILD SERVING

o o o

Tofu-Cheese Soufflé

1½ slices whole wheat bread
1 tbsp. butter or margarine
3 oz. sharp Cheddar cheese, grated
1 tbsp. chopped onion

3 oz. tofu, cut into ½-inch slices
¾ cup milk
2 eggs, beaten

Butter an ovenproof casserole. Spread bread with butter or margarine, break into several small pieces, and cover bottom of casserole with it. Then add grated cheese in one layer, the onion, and the tofu last. Combine milk and eggs, pour into casserole, and let stand for 1 hour. Preheat oven to 350°, place casserole in a larger pan of water, and bake for 45 minutes.

SERVES 2 TO 3

o o o

Tofu with Egg

2 tsp. butter or margarine
1 oz. tofu (2 tbsp.)
2 egg yolks
1 tsp. milk

In a skillet melt the butter or margarine, add tofu and mash, then sauté over medium heat until lightly brown. Beat egg yolks and milk together well, add to tofu, and scramble until eggs are cooked.

1 CHILD SERVING

o o o

Fried Tofu with Mushrooms

1 tbsp. peanut oil
1 tbsp. chopped onion
3 mushrooms, washed and
  sliced

2 tbsp. cooked peas
3 oz. tofu, cubed

Heat oil in a skillet and sauté onion in it until golden. Add mushrooms, peas, and tofu. Cook for 5 minutes over medium heat, stirring to brown tofu on all sides.

1 ADULT AND 1 CHILD SERVING

o o o

Mushroom Tofu Stroganoff

16 oz. tofu
1 tbsp. vegetable oil
1 clove garlic, minced
¾ lb. mushrooms, washed
    and sliced

¾ cup chicken stock
    (see page 280)
½ tsp. basil
Dash pepper
8 oz. plain yogurt
2 tbsp. flour

Drain tofu on paper towels and cut into ½-inch cubes. Heat oil in a skillet and fry tofu in it for 3 or 4 minutes, stirring to prevent sticking. Add garlic and mushrooms and cook for another 2 or 3 minutes until mushrooms are tender. Remove tofu and mushrooms, add chicken stock, basil, and pepper to skillet, and bring to a boil. Mix yogurt with flour and stir into stock, cooking until mixture bubbles. Cook for 1 minute more, then stir in tofu and mushrooms and heat through. Serve with noodles.

SERVES 4

o o o

Tofu-Rice Casserole

4 tsp. vegetable oil
2 tbsp. butter or margarine
1 medium onion, thinly
    sliced
1 cup cooked rice

12 oz. tofu, cut up
1 cup milk
½ cup bread crumbs
2 oz. Cheddar cheese,
    grated

Heat half the oil in a large skillet and add the butter or margarine. When melted, sauté onion until soft, then add rice and sauté for 2 minutes more. Gently stir in tofu, and sauté for another 2 minutes. Use remaining oil to grease an ovenproof dish, fill with tofu-rice mixture, and pour the cup of milk over it. Mix bread crumbs and grated cheese, sprinkle over the dish, and pop under preheated broiler until cheese is melted.

SERVES 2 TO 3

o o o

Vegetables Tofu

1 small sweet potato, peeled
   and cubed
1 small carrot, scrubbed and
   sliced
1 tbsp. butter or margarine
2 oz. tofu

Steam sweet potato and carrot together until tender. Mash well with butter or margarine and tofu. Serve immediately.

1 ADULT AND 1 CHILD SERVING

CHEESE AND EGGS

Cheese Enchiladas

Enchilada Sauce (see below)
Vegetable oil
1 package corn tortillas (12
   tortillas)

4 oz. shredded Cheddar
   cheese
4 oz. shredded jack cheese
1 green onion, chopped

(continued)

Make enchilada sauce. Heat oil in a frying pan and cook tortillas on both sides for a few minutes until soft. Drain on paper towels. Dip tortillas in enchilada sauce, lay on flat surface, and fill with 1 tablespoon each Cheddar and jack cheeses. Roll tortillas carefully and pin with toothpicks. Lay enchiladas side by side in a large ovenproof dish, cover with remaining sauce, and sprinkle with chopped onion and rest of cheese. Bake in preheated 350° oven for 10 to 15 minutes until cheese is melted. Serve immediately.

ENCHILADA SAUCE

1 cup tomato sauce (see page 283), or 8-oz. can tomato sauce
3 medium-size tomatoes, peeled and chopped

1 onion, peeled and chopped
4-oz. can diced mild green chiles
½ bunch fresh cilantro, washed and trimmed

Mix all ingredients in blender or food processor and pour into container large enough to dip tortillas.

SERVES 6 TO 8

○ ○ ○

Cheese and Lentil Loaf

½ lb. shredded Cheddar cheese
2 cups cooked drained lentils (see page 148)
½ small onion, peeled and chopped
⅛ tsp. black pepper
¼ tsp. thyme

1 cup soft bread crumbs, packed
1 egg, lightly beaten
1 tbsp. butter or margarine, melted
1 cup tomato sauce (see page 283)

Blend together shredded cheese, lentils, and onion, and add pepper and thyme. Stir in bread crumbs, beaten egg, and butter or margarine, and mix all ingredients thoroughly. Grease a loaf pan well, add mixture, and bake in preheated 325° oven for 45 minutes. Serve with heated tomato sauce.

SERVES 4

○ ○ ○

Cottage Cheese with Scrambled Egg

1 tbsp. cottage cheese*
1 egg
1 tsp. butter or margarine

Mix cottage cheese and egg in a bowl and beat well. Melt butter or margarine in a skillet and pour in mixture. Scramble over medium-low heat until cooked through.

1 CHILD SERVING

*Two tablespoons of cooked rice may be substituted for cottage cheese, if desired.

○ ○ ○

Quesadilla
(Tortilla with Cheese)

2 tbsp. grated jack or Cheddar cheese
1 small Mexican flour tortilla (see page 250)

Spread grated cheese on half the tortilla, fold, and press

down. Place on a baking sheet or foil in preheated 325° oven until cheese is melted.

Adults may add jalapeño peppers, salsa, guacamole, and sour cream, if desired.

1 CHILD SERVING

o o o

Ricotta Cheese Pancakes

3 eggs
1 cup ricotta or cottage
   cheese
2 tbsp. vegetable oil

2 tbsp. wheat germ
2 tbsp. flour

Combine all ingredients in a blender or food processor and mix until smooth. Pour 3-inch to 4-inch rounds of batter onto a greased and preheated griddle. Cook until bubbles form, turn, and continue to cook until brown.

SERVES 4

o o o

Asparagus Omelet

1 tbsp. butter or margarine
4 eggs, beaten
½ cup Swiss or Jarlsberg
   cheese, cut into small
   cubes

¾ cup cooked asparagus, cut
   into small pieces
½ cup tomatoes, peeled and
   cut up

Melt butter or margarine in an omelet or frying pan until bubbling. Pour eggs into pan and rotate until base is covered, pulling cooked egg gently inward and letting uncooked egg spread to the side. Add cheese, asparagus, and tomatoes and allow eggs to set. With a spatula, carefully fold omelet over, and cook for another minute or two, until cheese is melted. Slide omelet onto a warm plate and serve immediately.

SERVES 2

○ ○ ○

Egg Nest

½ cup puréed cooked fresh corn
1 tbsp. grated Parmesan cheese
1 egg

Put corn into a small individual ovenproof casserole and sprinkle with Parmesan cheese. Make a hollow in the corn and carefully break an egg into it. Bake in preheated 325° oven until set.

1 ADULT OR OLDER CHILD SERVING

○ ○ ○

Petite Omelet

1 tsp. butter or margarine
1 egg
1 oz. cooked chicken or
  ham, etc., cut into small
  cubes

1 small tomato, peeled and
  chopped
1 tsp. chopped parsley

Melt butter or margarine over medium heat in a small frying pan. Beat egg well in a bowl and mix in all other ingredients.

(continued)

When butter starts to bubble, pour egg mixture into center of pan and rotate to spread mixture, pulling cooked egg from sides and letting uncooked egg spread outside until omelet is set. Fold carefully with a spatula and slide onto a warm plate.

1 ADULT SERVING TO SHARE WITH 1 CHILD

o o o

Piselli con Uova
(Peas with Eggs)

2 tbsp. olive oil
1 small onion, peeled and
 chopped
2 cups canned plum
 tomatoes, puréed

½ tsp. basil
1 cup cooked fresh peas, or
 thawed frozen peas
4 eggs, individually beaten

In a large frying pan, heat oil and sauté onion in it until translucent. Add puréed tomatoes and basil, and simmer for 15 minutes, stirring occasionally. Then add peas and simmer for another 10 minutes. Add 1 beaten egg to pan and cook for 1 minute, stirring constantly. Do this 3 more times, allowing 1 minute for each egg to cook before adding the next. Serve immediately.

SERVES 2

○ ○ ○

Poached Egg with Spinach

1 bunch spinach (¾ to 1 lb.), washed and stems removed
2 eggs
6 orange segments, peeled and seeded

Cook spinach in a tightly covered pan, using only water remaining on the leaves, until tender. Remove from pan and chop fine. Poach eggs until whites are firm and place on beds of spinach in 2 bowls. Decorate around eggs with orange segments.

1 ADULT AND 1 CHILD SERVING

○ ○ ○

Scrambled Eggs with Peppers

1 tbsp. olive oil
1 medium-size onion,
  peeled and chopped
1 clove garlic, minced

1 medium-size bell pepper,
  washed, seeded, and
  diced
3 eggs, beaten

Heat oil in a skillet and in it gently sauté onion, garlic, and pepper until tender, about 10 minutes. Add beaten eggs and scramble over medium-low heat until firm. Serve with whole wheat bread.

1 ADULT AND 1 CHILD SERVING

○ ○ ○

Egg Custard

1 egg yolk, beaten
¼ cup milk
¼ tsp. vanilla extract

Blend egg yolk, milk, and vanilla. Pour mixture into a 4-oz.
ovenproof custard cup. Set cup in ovenproof pan, pour hot
water into pan until halfway up the side of the custard cup.
Bake in preheated 350° oven for 30 minutes, or until set.

1 CHILD SERVING

FISH

Haddock with Egg Butter

1 lb. fresh filleted haddock
Milk to cover
4 tbsp. butter or margarine
1 egg, hard-boiled and finely
  chopped

Place haddock in a saucepan, cover fish with milk, and put a
lid on pan. Slowly bring milk to a boil, reduce heat immediately, then simmer gently for 12 to 15 minutes. Meanwhile,
melt butter or margarine in a small saucepan, add chopped
egg, and mix. Remove fish from saucepan with a slotted
spoon, place on a hot platter, and cover with egg-butter mixture. Serve immediately with steamed carrots and potatoes.

SERVES 3 TO 4

○ ○ ○

Baked Haddock and Potatoes

3 large potatoes, scrubbed
   and sliced ⅛ inch thick
¼ cup melted butter or
   margarine
1 package frozen haddock
   (about 1 lb.), partially
   thawed

Juice of ½ lemon
½ tsp. paprika
½ tsp. dill

Generously grease an ovenproof casserole, add a layer of half the potato slices, and pour a little butter or margarine over them. Layer fish over potatoes, and sprinkle with lemon juice and half the paprika and dill. Top with remaining potatoes, cover with remaining butter or margarine, paprika, and dill. Cover and bake in preheated 375° oven for 1 hour, removing cover during the last 15 minutes and basting with butter from the casserole.

SERVES 3 TO 4

○ ○ ○

Fish with Fresh Tomato

4-oz. piece of skinned and filleted cod, halibut, or orange
   roughy
1 small ripe tomato
1 tsp. finely chopped parsley

Place fish in a saucepan of boiling water and simmer for 10 minutes, or until opaque. Remove with a slotted spoon and drain. Add tomato to boiling water for 2 minutes, then remove from water, peel, and chop well. Sprinkle fish with tomato and parsley, and serve with mashed potatoes.

1 ADULT AND 1 CHILD SERVING

o o o

Oven-Baked Fish

1 small fillet of fish (about 4
   oz.), skinned
1 egg

¼ cup milk
⅛ tsp. dill
½ tsp. chopped parsley

Cut fish into small pieces and place in a lightly oiled oven-proof dish. Beat together egg, milk, dill, and parsley, and pour over fish. Bake in preheated 350° oven for 15 to 20 minutes, or until fish flakes easily and is white in color.
    Serve with baked sweet potato and peas.

1 ADULT AND 1 CHILD SERVING

o o o

Fish and Rice Casserole

1½ cups rice (quick-cooking
   or basmati)
1 cup shredded carrot
⅓ cup thinly sliced celery
2 tbsp. butter or margarine
Grated peel of 1 lemon
1½ cups boiling chicken
   stock (preferably
   homemade, page 280)

1 lb. fresh sole, sea bass, or
   orange roughy, filleted
Juice of ½ lemon
Paprika

In a 12 × 8-inch baking dish, combine rice, carrot, celery, 1 tablespoon butter or margarine, lemon peel, and boiling chicken
stock. Cover with foil and bake in preheated 400° oven for 5
minutes. Remove from oven and stir. Arrange fish on top of
rice, sprinkle with lemon juice and paprika, and dot with remaining tablespoon of butter. Bake, covered, for 25 minutes,
or until fish flakes easily with fork.

SERVES 4

○ ○ ○

Simple Fish and Vegetables

2 oz. cod fillet, skinned
1 small carrot, scrubbed and thinly sliced
2 tbsp. chopped celery

Put fish, carrot, and celery in a small pan, and add enough
boiling water to cover. Simmer for 10 to 15 minutes, or until
fish and vegetables are cooked through. Pour off water, leaving just enough to mash with the fish and vegetables. Serve
with rice.

1 CHILD SERVING

o o o

Fiske Kaker
(Norwegian Fish Cakes)

1 lb. fresh haddock or cod,
   skinned, boned, and cut
   into pieces
1 tbsp. potato flour or
   cornstarch

1½ tsp. salt (necessary for
   the right texture)
⅛ tsp. ground nutmeg
1 cup milk
4 tbsp. butter

Put fish, flour, salt, and nutmeg in a food processor fitted
with metal blade. Process until fish has become a coarse purée, scraping down sides with spatula as necessary. With
processor running, add milk, 1 tablespoonful at a time, until
½ cup has been used. Then increase quantity to 2 or 3 tablespoonsful at a time until all milk has been used. Melt 2 tablespoons of butter in a frying pan over medium heat. Have
ready a bowl of water and a tablespoon. Moisten hand, dip
tablespoon into water, then into fish purée; with hand and
spoon form a round ball. Place fish cake in the frying pan and
flatten with a spatula or spoon until it is about ¾ inch thick.
Fry until brown, turn, and repeat on the other side until fish
cake is cooked through. Repeat until all purée is used up,
adding remaining butter as needed for frying.

SERVES 4

○ ○ ○

Creamy Halibut Bake

4 medium-size fresh halibut
  steaks
½ tsp. dill
½ onion, peeled and
  chopped
4 slices lemon

2 tbsp. butter or margarine
4 tomatoes, peeled and
  chopped
½ cup cream (or half-and-
  half)

Place halibut steaks side by side in an ovenproof casserole. Sprinkle with dill and onion. Place a slice of lemon on each steak, dot with butter or margarine, and cover with chopped tomatoes. Bake in preheated 375° oven, covered, for 20 to 25 minutes. Remove cover, add cream, and bake for another 10 minutes, basting occasionally.

SERVES 4

○ ○ ○

Poached Fish with Yogurt Sauce

1 quart water
1 small onion, peeled and
  quartered
6 whole black peppercorns
3 whole allspice

3 tbsp. lemon juice
1 bay leaf
1 tsp. salt
½ cup dry white wine
2 lbs. firm white fish, filleted
Yogurt Sauce (see below)
2 tbsp. chopped parsley

Place all ingredients except fish, yogurt sauce, and parsley in a large skillet and bring to a boil. Reduce heat and simmer, uncovered, for 30 minutes over low heat until flavors are blended. Add fish, cover, and continue to simmer for 15 to 20 minutes, until fish flakes easily when tested with a fork. Remove fish with a slotted spoon and drain well. Top with yogurt sauce. Garnish with parsley.

YOGURT SAUCE

1 cup plain yogurt
1 tbsp. cornstarch

2 tbsp. lemon juice
⅓ cup light mayonnaise

Mix yogurt with cornstarch in a small saucepan and bring to a low simmer, stirring with a wire whisk. Cook for 2 minutes, still stirring. Remove from heat. Beat lemon juice into yogurt mixture. Stir well. When cool, stir in the mayonnaise.

SERVES 4

○ ○ ○

Baked Potatoes with Salmon Sauce

4 medium-size potatoes
4 tbsp. butter or margarine
3 green onions, white parts
  only, finely chopped
½ cup mushrooms, washed
  and sliced

¼ cup all-purpose flour
½ tsp. marjoram
⅛ tsp. white pepper
Reserved liquid from can of
  salmon
2 cups milk
16-oz. can salmon, drained
  (reserve liquid)

Scrub potatoes and bake in preheated 350° oven for 1 hour, or until done. Meanwhile, melt butter or margarine in a saucepan, add onions and mushrooms, and sauté until tender. Add flour, marjoram, and pepper, mix well, then add the reserved liquid from the salmon. Slowly pour in milk, stirring constantly to mix, and cook over low heat until sauce is smooth and thickened. Break salmon into bite-size pieces, add to

sauce, and cook until thoroughly heated. Split open baked potatoes and spoon salmon sauce over them.

SERVES 4

o o o

Steamed Salmon Loaf

1 cup milk
1½ cups soft bread cubes
Two 16-oz. cans salmon
   with liquid
1 cup chopped celery
1 cup chopped onions
¼ cup chopped green
   pepper

4 eggs
2 tsp. grated lemon peel
1 tsp. lemon juice
½ tsp. paprika
½ tsp. thyme
½ tsp. black pepper

Scald milk, add bread cubes, and mix well. Flake salmon and
add it and liquid to milk. Add celery, onions, green pepper,
eggs, lemon peel and juice, paprika, thyme, and pepper to
pan and mix well. Oil an ovenproof loaf pan (about 9 × 5-
inch) and turn mixture into pan. Set loaf pan in a larger pan
half filled with hot water and bake in preheated 325° oven for
1½ hours. For easier cutting, let the salmon loaf sit for a while
before serving.

SERVES 6 TO 8

○ ○ ○

Baked Sea Bass Oriental

1 whole sea bass, cleaned
1 onion, sliced
3 slices lemon
Spicy Sweet Sauce (see
   below)

Place fish in an ovenproof dish and cover with onion, lemon, and the sauce. Bake in preheated 350° oven for 30 to 45 minutes, or until fish separates from the bones easily.

Check carefully to make sure *all* bones are removed before serving to children.

SPICY SWEET SAUCE

¼ cup soy sauce   ½ tsp. turmeric
3 small slices fresh ginger   ½ tsp. sugar
½ tsp. chili powder

Mix all ingredients together well before pouring over fish.

SERVES 3 TO 4

○ ○ ○

Seafood Salad

8 oz. vermicelli
¾ cup celery, thinly sliced
¼ cup chopped green or red
   pepper
3 hard-boiled eggs, chopped

2-oz. jar pimientos, chopped
   (optional)
Dressing (see below)
12 oz. cooked shrimp, crab,
   or filleted fish

Break vermicelli into bite-size pieces and cook in boiling water until tender (about 7 or 8 minutes). Drain and cool. Just before serving, mix all ingredients together in a large bowl with the dressing, but leave fish until last. Toss well and serve immediately.

DRESSING

½ cup light mayonnaise
½ cup buttermilk
1½ tbsp. lime or lemon juice
1 tsp. mixed Italian herbs

This is best made in advance. Combine all ingredients, mix well, and chill slightly before serving.

SERVES 4

○ ○ ○

Shrimp with Almond Yogurt Sauce

2 limes, thinly sliced
2 lbs. medium shrimp, peeled, cleaned, and deveined
⅓ cup very thinly slivered almonds
3 tbsp. butter or margarine
2 tbsp. minced onion

1 small clove garlic, minced
1 tsp. all-purpose flour
6 tbsp. vegetable or chicken stock (see page 281 or page 280)
½ cup plain yogurt

Line the bottom of a shallow ovenproof dish with sliced limes and arrange shrimp over them. Sprinkle with 1 tablespoon slivered almonds and put under preheated broiler for 6 minutes, turning once after 3 minutes. Transfer to a serving platter and keep warm. Melt butter or margarine in a saucepan, add remaining almonds, onion, and garlic. Sauté until onion is golden, then stir in flour, add stock, and continue to cook over low to medium heat until sauce has thickened. Remove from heat and stir in yogurt until creamy and well blended. Sauce may be served over shrimp or on the side.

SERVES 4

○ ○ ○

Shrimp and Okra Stew

3 tbsp. vegetable oil
1 medium-size onion, chopped
1 lb. fresh or frozen okra, sliced thin
4 medium-size tomatoes, blanched and peeled

2 ripe plantains (or bananas), cubed
½ lb. shrimp
2 to 3 cups broth (chicken, fish, or vegetable) (see pages 280–282)
Juice of a lime (or lemon)

Heat oil in a large pot, add onion, and sauté until glazed. Add okra, tomatoes, and plantains (or bananas). Simmer for 5 minutes, stirring occasionally, then add shrimp, broth, and lime (or lemon) juice. Bring stew to a boil, immediately reduce heat, and simmer for 30 minutes, covered. Stir frequently but gently to prevent sticking.

A little salt or other seasonings, such as dill, garlic, pepper, etc., may be added for adults. Serve over rice.

SERVES 4

○ ○ ○

Sole Meunière

¼ tsp. salt
⅛ tsp. white pepper
¼ cup flour
1 lb. fresh fillet of sole

¼ pound (1 stick) butter or margarine, divided in half
2 tbsp. fresh lime or lemon juice
1 tbsp. finely chopped parsley

Combine salt and pepper with flour and coat fish lightly with the mixture. Melt half the butter or margarine in a frying pan until bubbly and sauté fish in it, carefully turning once when the first side is browned. Fish is cooked when white and flaky. Remove to a hot platter.

Clean pan, add remaining butter or margarine, lime or lemon juice, and parsley, and heat gently until butter is melted and ingredients are mixed. Remove from heat and pour over fish. Serve immediately.

SERVES 3 TO 4

○ ○ ○

Calamari

3 tbsp. olive or safflower oil
2 large cloves garlic, crushed
1 onion, peeled and sliced thin
1 stalk celery, chopped
12 mushrooms, washed and sliced

2 tomatoes, peeled and chopped
1½ cups tomato sauce (see page 283)
1 tsp. tarragon
1 lb. squid, cleaned and cut up

Heat oil in a large pan and in it cook garlic, onion, and celery until tender. Add mushrooms, tomatoes, tomato sauce, and tarragon, and continue cooking over medium heat for 10 minutes, stirring occasionally to prevent sticking. Add squid to sauce, mix well, and bring mixture to a boil. Reduce heat immediately and simmer for 10 minutes. (Important: Do not overcook squid, as it will become tough.) Serve with rice and a green salad.

SERVES 4

o o o

Stir-Fried Squid with Snow Peas

MARINADE

½-inch piece fresh ginger,
   peeled and grated

Juice of 1 lime
1 tbsp. soy sauce

1 lb. squid,* cleaned and
   cut up
6 tbsp. peanut oil
24 Chinese snow peas,
   washed and trimmed

12 mushrooms, washed
   and sliced
½ tsp. arrowroot

Combine ingredients for marinade, cut squid into 1 × ½-inch pieces, and marinate for 15 minutes. Heat oil in a wok or heavy frying pan until very hot, then add squid, snow peas, and mushrooms. Stir-fry for approximately 3 minutes until squid is opaque and snow peas are bright green. Remove from wok to a heated plate. Add arrowroot to marinade, put in wok, and stir well until heated through to make a sauce. Pour over squid and serve immediately with rice.

SERVES 3 TO 4

*Abalone, sea bass, or halibut may be substituted for squid, if desired.

o o o

Broiled Sturgeon

1 lb. sturgeon, skinned and   2 tbsp. lemon juice
   boned   2 tbsp. chopped fresh dill
3 tbsp. olive oil   Paprika

Cut fish into 1½-inch chunks and marinate in mixture of oil, lemon, and dill for 20 minutes. Drain fish and reserve marinade. Place fish in a shallow heatproof dish, sprinkle with paprika, and place under preheated broiler for 5 minutes, basting frequently with marinade. Turn and broil for 5 more minutes, continuing to baste. Fish is cooked when it becomes white and flaky.

SERVES 3 TO 4

o o o

Tuna Fish Casserole

2 cups wide egg noodles
2 cups Cheese Sauce (see below)
Two 6½-oz. cans white or light tuna, drained and flaked

Cook noodles as directed on package. Meanwhile, make the cheese sauce. Preheat oven to 350° and mix noodles, cheese sauce, and tuna together in an ovenproof dish. Bake for 20 to 30 minutes.

CHEESE SAUCE

3 tbsp. butter or margarine   4 oz. medium-sharp
3 tbsp. flour   Cheddar cheese, grated
10 oz. milk   Dash white pepper

(continued)

Melt butter or margarine over *very low heat* until melted. Add flour and stir gently with a wooden spoon. Add milk and bring slowly to a boil, stirring constantly to prevent lumpiness. Reduce heat and simmer for no more than 2 to 3 minutes. Add cheese and pepper, and continue stirring until cheese is melted.

SERVES 3 TO 4

o o o

Tuna Melt

6-oz. can tuna, packed in
  water
1 tbsp. light mayonnaise
  (or 1 tbsp. regular
  mayonnaise mixed with 1
  tbsp. plain yogurt)

½ tsp. dill
4 slices whole wheat bread
2 oz. mozzarella cheese,
  grated

Mix tuna, mayonnaise, and dill. Spread on each slice of bread, top with cheese, and broil until cheese melts.

SERVES 4

POULTRY

Chicken Breasts with Lime Butter

4 boneless chicken breasts,
   skinned
1 egg, beaten
½ cup bread crumbs
2 tbsp. olive oil

Juice of 1 lime
¼ pound (1 stick) butter or
   margarine
1 tsp. minced fresh chives
½ tsp. dill

Place chicken breasts between two pieces of wax paper and pound until very thin. (A rolling pin or a wooden potato masher works well.) Dip chicken in beaten egg, then in bread crumbs. Heat oil in a skillet and sauté chicken in it over medium heat for 2 to 3 minutes on each side, or until meat is white throughout. Transfer to a warm platter. Drain remaining oil from skillet, add lime juice, and heat over low flame until it bubbles. Add butter or margarine and stir until mixture becomes opaque and thickened. Stir in chives and dill. Spoon sauce over chicken and serve immediately.

SERVES 4

○ ○ ○

Boned Chicken Chinese Style

1 boned, skinned chicken
   breast, sliced thin and cut
   into bite-size pieces
½ cup soy sauce
2 tbsp. port or sherry
1 slice lemon
2 cloves garlic, peeled and
   split in half
2 slices fresh ginger

1 tbsp. safflower or
   peanut oil
1 cup bean sprouts, washed
1 cup mushrooms, washed
   and sliced
1 onion, peeled and sliced
2 cups Chinese snow peas,
   washed and trimmed
1 tsp. cornstarch or
   arrowroot

Marinate chicken breast in mixture of soy sauce, port or
sherry, lemon, garlic, and ginger for at least 1 hour. Drain
chicken and save marinade. Heat oil in a wok over medium-
high heat. Throw in sprouts, mushrooms, onion, and snow
peas, and stir-fry for 2 to 3 minutes. Remove vegetables and
add a little more oil, if necessary, to cook chicken. Stir-fry
chicken for 5 to 7 minutes, or until cooked through. Remove
chicken and set aside with vegetables. Mix cornstarch or arrowroot with marinade, first removing lemon, ginger, and
garlic, and stir well. Throw chicken and vegetables back into
wok, add marinade, and mix together over high heat. Serve
immediately with rice.

SERVES 2

o o o

Cuban Chicken

1 onion, peeled and
  quartered
1 green pepper, washed,
  seeded, and quartered
1 chicken, washed, skinned,
  and cut into serving
  pieces
1 small can tomato sauce
1 small jar green olives,
  drained
1 small jar pimientos, cut
  into 1-inch squares

1 handful raisins
½ bottle Cuban or California
  white wine
1½ tbsp. cumin
1 tsp. garlic salt
4 potatoes, quartered
4 carrots, scrubbed and cut
  into thirds

Place onion and pepper in blender or food processor, using chopping blade, and chop fine. Put chicken pieces into a large pot, add onion, green pepper, and all other ingredients except potatoes and carrots. Bring to a boil, reduce heat, and simmer for 1½ hours. Add potatoes and carrots and return to heat for ½ hour more, or until vegetables are cooked through.

SERVES 4

o o o

Chicken Fricassee

1 whole stewing chicken,
  skinned
1 carrot, scrubbed
1 onion, peeled
2 stalks celery, washed

1 tsp. salt
½ tsp. white pepper
White sauce (see page 284)
3 tbsp. chopped parsley

(continued)

Clean chicken well, put in a heavy pot, and cover with water. Add carrot, onion, celery, and salt and pepper. Bring to a boil, reduce heat, and simmer for 1 hour, or until chicken falls from the bones. Remove chicken from pot with tongs, let cool, then remove meat and discard skin and bones. Strain broth through a sieve, saving some to use for white sauce and discarding carrot, onion, and celery. Make white sauce according to recipe, using broth from the chicken. Cut chicken into bite-size pieces, add to white sauce, heat thoroughly, and pour fricassee into a heated serving dish. Dress with chopped parsley and serve with cauliflower, carrots, and buttered potatoes.

SERVES 4

o o o

Pineapple Chicken Supreme

1 chicken breast, boned,
  skinned, and pounded flat
2 tbsp. flour
¼ cup oil
¼ cup fresh or canned
  pineapple juice
¼ cup orange juice

¼ cup tomato juice
Juice of ¼ lemon
1 tsp. cornstarch
1 tbsp. water
⅓ cup diced fresh or canned
  pineapple

Cut chicken breast into 1-inch pieces and dredge in flour. Heat oil in a wok or heavy skillet. When oil is hot, quickly stir-fry chicken until cooked (about 3 minutes), remove, and drain on paper towels. Combine all the juices and bring to a boil in wok. Dissolve cornstarch in water, stir into juices, return to a boil, and cook 1 minute, or until mixture is thick and clear. Add chicken and pineapple, stir well, and serve immediately.

Purée or cut up well for infants.

1 ADULT AND 1 CHILD SERVING

○ ○ ○

Roast Chicken in Tomato Sauce

1 roasting chicken, washed (or chicken parts)
2 cups tomato sauce (see page 283)

Preheat oven to 375°, place chicken in roasting pan breast side down, and cook for 1 hour. Remove chicken from pan. Drain off excess fat, add tomato sauce to pan, and stir, scraping brown glaze from bottom of pan. Turn chicken breast side up; replace in pan, continue cooking for another 30 minutes, and baste with sauce. Serve with the tomato sauce over rice.

SERVES 4

○ ○ ○

Baked Chicken with Tarragon

1 roasting chicken
1 cup dry white wine
1 tsp. tarragon
Dash white pepper

Wash and dry chicken and place in an ovenproof dish. Pour wine over chicken, rub with tarragon and pepper, and bake in preheated 350° oven for 1½ hours, or until juices run clear. For a crisper skin and the best flavor, baste with wine-meat juices occasionally. (The alcohol in the wine evaporates during cooking.)

SERVES 4 TO 5

o o o

Groundnut Chicken Stew

4 tbsp. vegetable oil
1 medium-size onion,
   peeled and chopped
1 stewing chicken, washed,
   skinned, and cut into
   serving pieces
4 medium-size tomatoes,
   peeled and chopped

2 cups chicken stock
   (see page 280)
½ tsp. thyme
½ cup peanut butter
6-oz. can tomato paste
3 hard-boiled eggs
2 tbsp. chopped parsley

In a large heavy pot heat oil and lightly sauté onion in it. Add chicken and brown on both sides. Add tomatoes, stock, and thyme, mix well, and bring to a boil. Reduce heat and simmer, covered, for 15 minutes. Remove enough liquid from pot to mix with peanut butter and tomato paste to make a gravy, combine well, return to pot, and simmer chicken for 45 minutes more. Garnished with sliced hard-boiled eggs and parsley, serve stew over boiled rice.

SERVES 4 TO 5

MEATS

Baked Ham in Vegetable Juice

1 lb. canned ham
6-oz. can V-8 or similar vegetable juice

Place ham in a small ovenproof dish and pour vegetable juice over it. Bake in preheated 350° oven for 30 minutes, or until thoroughly heated.

SERVES 4

○ ○ ○

Scalloped Potatoes with Ham

1 cup thinly sliced potatoes
2 slices ham, cut into 1-inch
   pieces
¾ cup milk
2 tbsp. butter or margarine

Grease an ovenproof dish and preheat oven to 350°. Layer potatoes and ham in dish, bring milk to a boil and add butter or margarine, and pour over potatoes and ham. Cover dish and bake for 1 hour, or until potatoes are tender.

SERVES 2 TO 3

o o o

Baby Pasta with Meat Sauce

3 tbsp. stelline (small star-shaped macaroni)
1 tbsp. finely chopped onion
1 tsp. olive oil

3 tbsp. lean ground beef or turkey
3 tbsp. tomato sauce (see page 283), or 1 tbsp. tomato paste mixed with 2 tbsp. water

Cook stelline according to directions on package. In a skillet sauté onion in olive oil until tender, add crumbled ground meat, and cook over low heat until browned. Add tomato sauce, mix well with meat, and simmer for 1 or 2 minutes to develop flavor. Stir mixture into cooked stelline and serve.

1 OR 2 INFANT SERVINGS

o o o

Beef, Bean, and Macaroni Casserole

½ lb. lean ground beef
1 small onion, peeled and chopped
2 cups canned tomatoes (reserve liquid), chopped
1 cup cooked kidney beans (see page 146; reserve liquid)

1 cup cooked elbow macaroni
½ tsp. basil
½ tsp. oregano
½ tsp. chili powder

In a large skillet, brown beef and onion. Drain off fat. If necessary, add water to combined tomato and bean liquid to equal 1 cup, and add to skillet with tomatoes, kidney beans, macaroni, and seasonings. Cover and simmer for approximately 10 minutes. Stir occasionally to prevent sticking; if necessary, add more liquid during cooking.

SERVES 4

o o o

Cabbage Rolls

1 cabbage
½ onion, peeled and
    chopped
1 tbsp. cooking oil
½ lb. lean ground beef
    or turkey
¼ cup uncooked rice

1 tbsp. parsley, finely
    chopped
1 cup tomato sauce (see
    page 283)
Sufficient chicken or
    vegetable stock or broth to
    cover rolls (see page 280
    or page 281)

Remove any torn outer leaves from cabbage, then cut out core with sharp knife, being careful to keep cabbage whole. Place cabbage, base down, in a large pot, cover with boiling water, and blanch for 5 minutes. Remove, drain, and, when cool, separate leaves, using 8 of the best large outer leaves for the rolls. In a skillet gently sauté onion in oil until soft, then mix in a large bowl with uncooked meat, rice, parsley, and ½ cup tomato sauce. Put 1 large tablespoon of filling into each leaf and fold, envelope style, making sure it is "sealed." Place extra cabbage leaves on the bottom of a large flameproof pan, put cabbage rolls on top of leaves, seam side down, and cover with stock. Weight rolls down with a heavy plate, cover pan, and simmer for 1¼ hours. Serve with remainder of the tomato sauce, or make a brown sauce if desired.

SERVES 4

o o o

Halloween Stew (in a Pumpkin)

2 onions, peeled and
chopped
2 cloves garlic, minced
1½ lbs. stewing beef, cubed
1 tbsp. vegetable oil
2 green peppers, diced
4 tomatoes, peeled and
diced
2 white potatoes, peeled and
diced
2 sweet potatoes, peeled
and diced

1 cup sweet corn
1 cup diced pumpkin
(optional)
½ cup diced fresh peaches
(optional)
Salt and pepper to taste
4 cups stock or water
1 pumpkin, 15 inches in
diameter, for serving

In a large pot sauté onions, garlic, and beef in oil until meat
is browned and onions are tender. Add all remaining ingredients except pumpkin, bring to a boil, reduce heat, and simmer
until meat is tender (1½ to 2 hours). While stew is cooking,
cut a lid-size piece from top of pumpkin, remove seeds and
pulp, but leave firm flesh intact. Preheat oven to 375° and
steam pumpkin, with lid alongside, in ovenproof dish with 2
inches of water until tender but still firm (about 1 hour). Set
pumpkin in a serving dish, carefully fill with hot stew, and
replace the lid. To serve, spoon out stew and carefully cut out
inside of pumpkin flesh to serve with stew, if desired.

SERVES 4 ADULTS AND 4 CHILDREN

o o o

Meatballs

5 oz. ground sirloin or
   turkey
3 tbsp. bread crumbs
2 tbsp. grated onion

4 tbsp. water
Dash salt (optional)
1 tbsp. vegetable oil

In a mixing bowl put meat, bread crumbs, onion, and water
(plus salt, if desired), and mix well. Shape into 1-inch meatballs, and fry in a little oil over low heat until cooked through.

1 ADULT AND 1 CHILD SERVING

o o o

Meat Cakes

1 lb. lean or extra-lean
   ground beef
1 egg
1 tbsp. bread crumbs
A little milk, if necessary

Mix all ingredients thoroughly, using milk if necessary to hold
mixture together. For each meat cake take 1 tablespoonful of
meat and pat into a 2-inch round. Cook in a skillet over medium heat until meat is cooked through and all redness is
gone.

MAKES 12 MEAT CAKES (MAY BE FROZEN AND REHEATED LATER)

○ ○ ○

Shepherd's Pie

1 lb. lean ground beef or
   lamb
1 medium onion, peeled and
   chopped
1 cup stewed tomatoes, or 2
   or 3 fresh tomatoes,
   peeled and chopped

1 tbsp. finely chopped
   parsley
Dash Worcestershire sauce
¼ tsp. ground pepper
4 cups hot mashed potatoes
1 tbsp. butter or margarine

Slowly brown ground meat and onion until meat is cooked
and crumbly and onion is tender (add oil only if fat from meat
is insufficient). Stir in tomatoes, parsley, Worcestershire
sauce, and pepper; mix and heat thoroughly. Transfer mixture
to a heatproof dish, top with hot mashed potatoes, and dot
with butter or margarine. Put under preheated broiler and
cook for 8 to 10 minutes, or until potato is golden and crisp.

SERVES 4

○ ○ ○

Zucchini Beef Skillet

1 lb. lean ground beef
1 small onion, peeled and
   chopped
1 lb. zucchini, washed and
   sliced

1 clove garlic, minced
16-oz. can whole tomatoes
Dash pepper
2 tsp. oregano

In large skillet brown ground beef with onion (add oil only if
fat from meat is insufficient). Drain off fat. Add all remaining
ingredients and stir. Cover and simmer for 15 minutes.

SERVES 4

○ ○ ○

Arabian Stew

2 tbsp. olive oil
1 medium-size onion,
    peeled and chopped
1 lb. stewing lamb, cut into
    1-inch cubes
1 cup peeled and chopped
    tomatoes

1 tbsp. chopped fresh mint
    leaves
Salt and pepper
4 cups hot water
1 cup cooked vermicelli

Heat oil in a large saucepan and sauté onion until golden brown, add meat, and brown on all sides. Add tomatoes, mint, and seasonings, stir well, and cover with hot water. Bring to a boil and simmer for 1 hour, covered, stirring occasionally. Season to taste. Add cooked vermicelli, heat through, and serve immediately.

Purée or shred meat for infants.

SERVES 4

○ ○ ○

Roast Lamb and Potatoes

1 leg of lamb
Pepper and rosemary
2 cloves garlic, sliced
6 medium-size potatoes,
    peeled and halved
    lengthwise

1 tbsp. flour
2 cups vegetable stock (see
    page 281) or water

Rub lamb with pepper and rosemary, make small slits diagonally in skin, and insert garlic slices. Place lamb in a roasting pan and cook in preheated 325° oven for 25 to 30 minutes per pound. Baste occasionally with juices, and add potatoes around the meat approximately 1½ hours before lamb is done. Turn potatoes after 45 minutes to finish browning.

To make pan gravy, remove lamb and potatoes and place on a hot platter. Remove excess fat from roasting pan, leaving 1 or 2 tablespoons. Take pan off heat, add flour to drippings, and mix with a wooden spoon, scraping pan well. Return pan to low to medium heat, add vegetable stock or water, and bring to a boil. Reduce heat and simmer, stirring to prevent burning, until gravy is well blended and thickened.

Purée or finely chop meat for infants and toddlers.

SERVES 6 TO 8

o o o

Leftover Lamb with Beans

Lean cooked lamb and lamb
   shank
5 cups vegetable stock (see
   page 281) or water

1 onion, peeled and
   quartered
1 cup small dried white
   beans
1 bay leaf
Leftover vegetables

Cut meat from leftover leg of lamb, trim off fat, and put meat and bone in a large heavy pan. Cover with stock or water, add onion, beans, and bay leaf, and bring to a boil over medium heat. Reduce heat and simmer for 2 hours. Remove bone from pan. Add leftover vegetables (especially potatoes, carrots, and peas) and reheat.

For adults, ½ cup of red wine and other seasonings may be added to stew, if desired.

SERVES 4

o o o

Norwegian Lamb and Cabbage

2 lbs. lean lamb, cut into
    1-inch cubes
2 heads cabbage, washed
    and sliced
½ tsp. salt

2 tbsp. flour
2 cups water
Handful whole
    peppercorns, tied in
    cheesecloth

Layer lamb and cabbage in a heavy pan, starting with a layer of meat. Sprinkle a little salt and flour between each layer. Add water and peppercorns, cover pan, and simmer on top of stove for 2 to 3 hours, frequently stirring to prevent burning and to mix in peppercorn flavor. Serve with boiled potatoes.

For infants, purée or finely chop meat and cabbage.

SERVES 6 TO 8

GRAINS AND PASTA

Cooked Barley

1 tbsp. barley
2 cups water

Bring barley and water to a boil in a saucepan. Reduce heat, cover, and simmer for 1½ hours or until barley is tender.

Small amounts (up to 2 ounces or so) of cooked meat and/ or vegetables may be added to the barley, if desired. Heat through for a minute or two before serving.

SERVES 1

o o o

Bulgur Pilaf

4 tbsp. butter or margarine
1 small onion, peeled and
   minced
1 coil vermicelli, broken into
   pieces

1 cup cracked wheat
   (bulgur)
2½ cups chicken stock (see
   page 280)

Melt butter or margarine in a pan, add onion and vermicelli, and brown lightly. Add cracked wheat and chicken stock, and bring to a boil. Stir well to mix, cover, reduce heat, and simmer for 20 minutes. Remove from heat and let stand for 5 minutes. Fluff with fork before serving.

SERVES 4

o o o

Cornmeal Mush

2 cups water
½ cup cornmeal

Bring 1½ cups of water to a boil over medium heat. Mix remaining water with cornmeal and add to boiling water, stirring constantly. Cook over low heat for 5 minutes, stirring continually until ready.

SERVES 4

○ ○ ○

Millet Cereal

½ cup millet, well rinsed
¼ cup powdered skim milk
1½ cups water

Combine ingredients in a heavy pan, bring to a boil, reduce heat, and simmer for 10 minutes, stirring occasionally. Remove pan from heat, cover, and let stand for 30 minutes.

SERVES 4

○ ○ ○

Basmati Rice

1 cup basmati (Indian) rice
2 cups water
1 tbsp. butter or margarine

Pick impurities out of rice and wash well under cold water, using a fine sieve. Move rice around with hands until water runs clear. Bring 2 cups water to a boil, add rice, and stir with a fork. Reduce heat, cover, and cook for 10 minutes. Remove from heat and let stand for 10 more minutes. Add butter or margarine and fluff rice with fork before serving.

SERVES 3

o o o

Rice with Cheese

1 cup cooked rice
½ cup milk
½ cup grated Parmesan or Romano cheese

Put rice in a small saucepan and add a little milk. Over medium heat alternately add grated cheese and remaining milk, stirring constantly. Continue to simmer for a few minutes until the flavors are blended.

1 ADULT AND 1 CHILD SERVING

o o o

Italian Rice and Avocado Salad

½ cup rice
1¼ cups water, in all
2 medium-size zucchini, washed and coarsely grated
1 lb. sweet Italian sausages
1 tbsp. vegetable oil

2 avocados, peeled, pitted, and sliced
1 large tomato, peeled and chopped
¾ cup chopped parsley
Italian Dressing (see below)

Cook ½ cup rice in 1 cup water in a medium-size pan. When done, stir in zucchini, cover, and set aside. Pierce sausages with a fork and place in a skillet with ¼ cup water, cover, and simmer for 10 minutes. Drain off liquid. Add oil to skillet and cook sausages over medium-low heat, tossing occasionally, for 8 minutes, or until cooked through and browned. Drain sausages, then halve and cut into strips lengthwise. Combine with rice-zucchini mixture, add avocados, tomato, and parsley, and toss with Italian dressing.

ITALIAN DRESSING

¼ cup vinegar
2 tsp. oregano
1 tsp. rosemary
¼ tsp. salt

⅛ tsp. black pepper
1 medium-size clove garlic,
   crushed
¼ cup olive oil

Combine all ingredients except olive oil in a blender or food processor and blend well. With machine at low speed, gradually add olive oil and continue blending until thoroughly mixed. Makes ⅔ cup of dressing.

SERVES 4

o o o

Rice Royal

1 cup uncooked rice
2 tbsp. butter or margarine
1½ cups grated Cheddar
   cheese
1 cup finely chopped parsley

Cook rice. Add butter or margarine, grated cheese, and parsley while rice is still hot. Stir to mix well and serve immediately.

SERVES 4

○ ○ ○

Tabbouleh Salad

¼ cup finely cracked wheat (bulgur)
½ cup minced parsley
1 cup peeled, seeded, and chopped tomatoes
¼ cup chopped fresh mint

¼ cup lemon juice
2 tbsp. green onion, finely chopped
¼ cup olive oil
Romaine lettuce

Soak cracked wheat for 10 minutes in enough water to cover. Drain and squeeze as dry as possible in a clean white towel. Place cracked wheat in a large bowl. Add all ingredients except oil and lettuce and mix well. Let stand for 30 minutes to allow flavors to blend, then add oil, mixing and tossing lightly. Serve on a bed of romaine lettuce.

SERVES 4 TO 6

○ ○ ○

Beans and Broccoli with Stars

2 tbsp. stelline (cooked according to directions on package)
2 tbsp. small dried white beans, cooked (see page 146)

½ cup tomato sauce (see page 283) or canned
1 small broccoli floret, steamed and diced

Combine stelline (star-shaped pasta) with beans and tomato sauce in a small pan. Mix and cook over low heat for 5 minutes, then add broccoli to heat through (1 minute).

1 CHILD SERVING

o o o

Cottage Cheese and Noodle Casserole

8 oz. broad noodles
1 egg, lightly beaten
2 cups small-curd cottage
   cheese

¼ cup melted butter or
   margarine
¼ cup bread crumbs

Cook noodles according to directions on package and drain. Mix lightly beaten egg into cottage cheese. Grease an oven-proof dish, place in it a layer of noodles followed by the cottage cheese, and top with remaining noodles. Mix butter or margarine and bread crumbs together and cover noodles with mixture. Bake in preheated 375° oven for 30 minutes.

SERVES 2 TO 3

o o o

Macaroni Broccoli Sauté

2 cups cooked broccoli
4 tbsp. olive oil
1 clove garlic, peeled and
   crushed

¼ cup diced pimiento
1 cup small cooked macaroni

Finely chop broccoli. In a skillet heat oil and add garlic and pimiento. Mix and cook for 30 seconds, then add cooked macaroni and broccoli. Cook over low heat until flavors are well blended and ingredients are heated through.

1 ADULT AND 1 CHILD SERVING

○ ○ ○

Macaroni Marinara

⅓ cup cooked tubettini (or other small pasta)
¼ cup marinara sauce (see page 283)
1 small cooked potato, diced

Mix ingredients together in a small pan and simmer for 2 to 3 minutes.

1 OR 2 CHILD SERVINGS

○ ○ ○

Macaroni Salad

1 cup small macaroni
1 cup peeled and thinly
  sliced cucumber
1 cup diced tomatoes
½ cup chopped celery
¼ cup chopped green
  pepper
6½-oz. can tuna, shredded
  (optional)

1 tsp. dill
½ cup light mayonnaise
¼ cup ready-made Italian
  dressing
Lettuce for garnish
1 hard-boiled egg, sliced

Cook, drain, and chill macaroni. Mix together all ingredients (including shredded tuna if desired) except lettuce and egg until blended. Arrange washed lettuce leaves in a salad bowl, covering base and sides. Add macaroni salad and decorate with hard-boiled egg slices. Chill until ready to serve.

SERVES 4

o o o

Baked Mostaccioli

½ onion, peeled and
   chopped
1 clove garlic, minced
1 tbsp. olive oil
4 oz. ground beef
1 tbsp. chopped parsley

2 cups tomato sauce (see
   page 283) or canned
8 oz. mostaccioli pasta
1 cup Cheddar cheese,
   thinly sliced or grated

In a skillet, cook onion and garlic in oil until tender and drain. In same skillet brown beef with parsley until crumbly, and drain off any excess fat. Add tomato sauce, bring to a boil, reduce heat, and simmer for 15 minutes, stirring occasionally. Meanwhile, cook pasta until tender, drain well, and place in a heatproof casserole. When meat sauce is ready, pour over pasta and mix well. Cover completely with sliced or grated cheese and pop under preheated broiler until cheese is melted and bubbling.

SERVES 2 TO 3

o o o

Pasta and Chick-peas

2 cups canned peeled Italian
   tomatoes, crushed
3 tbsp. olive oil
1 tbsp. chopped parsley
¼ tsp. basil

1 clove garlic, peeled
⅛ tsp. pepper
1 cup cooked chick-peas
   (garbanzo beans)
1 cup cooked ditalini

Combine all ingredients except chick-peas and ditalini in a saucepan, bring to a boil, and simmer for 20 minutes. Remove garlic clove, add chick-peas and ditalini, and simmer for 1 or 2 minutes, stirring until well blended and heated through.

SERVES 2 TO 3

○ ○ ○

Pasta e Fagioli
(Macaroni and Beans)

1 tsp. olive oil
Small clove garlic, peeled
⅓ cup canned Italian plum
   tomatoes, chopped
¼ tsp. oregano

Pinch pepper
4 tbsp. cooked ditalini or
   small elbow macaroni
2 tbsp. small dried white
   beans, cooked (see page
   146)

Heat oil in a pan and cook garlic clove for 1 minute. Add tomatoes, oregano, and pepper, and simmer for 5 minutes. Remove garlic. Add pasta and beans to the sauce and simmer for 5 more minutes, stirring occasionally to blend.

1 CHILD SERVING

○ ○ ○

Pasta with Peas

¼ onion, finely chopped
2 tbsp. olive oil
½ cup canned Italian
   tomatoes, sieved or
   puréed

Pinch each oregano and
   pepper
½ cup cooked tubettini (or
   other small pasta)
½ cup fresh or frozen small
   peas

Sauté onion in oil in a medium-size pan until tender. Add tomatoes and seasonings, bring to a boil, reduce heat, and simmer for 5 minutes. Add tubettini and peas, stir gently, and continue to simmer for another 5 minutes.

1 ADULT AND 1 CHILD SERVING

○ ○ ○

Stelline with Cottage Cheese

3 tbsp. stelline (or other small pasta)
1 tbsp. butter or margarine, melted
4 tbsp. small-curd cottage cheese

Cook pasta according to directions on package, drain, and add melted butter or margarine. Add cottage cheese and toss well.

1 CHILD SERVING

SOUPS

Cream of Broccoli Soup

2 lbs. cooked and cooled
  broccoli (stems are good
  for soup)
2 cups vegetable or chicken
  stock (see page 281 or
  page 280)

2 cups milk
4 tbsp. butter or margarine
½ tsp. garlic powder
¼ tsp. white pepper

Put broccoli in a food processor or blender with some of the stock. Purée, pour mixture into a saucepan, and add all other ingredients. Heat over very low heat, stirring well until heated through.

SERVES 4 TO 6

o o o

Celery Soup

1 bunch celery, tops
  included, washed
4 leeks, white parts only,
  well washed
3 potatoes, peeled

1½ quarts water
5 mushrooms, washed
¼ cup *tamari* or soy sauce
1 tsp. celery salt
⅛ tsp. each thyme and basil

Slice vegetables thin. Place all vegetables except mushrooms in a pot with 1½ quarts of water and bring to a boil. Add sauce and seasonings, cover, reduce heat, and simmer for 10 minutes. In a blender or food processor, purée mixture in batches. Return purée to the pot, add sliced mushrooms, and simmer for 30 minutes. Stir frequently and make sure the soup does not scorch.

SERVES 6

o o o

Cold Cream of Avocado Soup

3 ripe avocados, peeled,
  pitted, and diced
1 cup chicken stock (see
  page 280)
2 tsp. lime or lemon juice

1 clove garlic, peeled and
  minced
½ tsp. salt
1 cup half-and-half

Combine avocados and chicken stock in a blender or food processor, and purée until smooth. Add lime or lemon juice, garlic, and salt, and continue to blend. Pour into a bowl and stir in half-and-half or cream. Chill well before serving.

SERVES 2

o o o

Cream of Tomato Soup

2 tbsp. butter or margarine
½ onion, peeled and
  chopped
1 medium-size potato,
  peeled and cubed
1½ cups chicken stock (see
  page 280)

5 ripe tomatoes, peeled and
  chopped
1½ cups milk
½ cup cooked tiny macaroni
  (optional)
2 hard-boiled eggs, halved
  (optional)

(continued)

Melt butter or margarine in a heavy pot and sauté onion and potato in it for 3 minutes, or until onion is glazed. Add chicken stock to pot, bring to a boil, reduce heat, and simmer until potato is tender (between 5 and 10 minutes). Place tomatoes in a food processor or blender, add broth and potato, and purée until smooth. Return soup to pot, add milk, and heat thoroughly but *do not allow to boil*. Stir in macaroni, if desired, and keep over low heat until warmed. Put egg halves in bowls and ladle soup over.

Small pieces of steamed broccoli, cauliflower, or squash may also be added for variety.

SERVES 4

o o o

Karin's Health Soup

1 cup soybeans, soaked
  overnight
4 cups vegetable or chicken
  stock (see page 281 or
  page 280)

3 potatoes, peeled and diced
½ cabbage, diced
2 cups chopped broccoli
Salt and pepper

Bring soybeans to a boil in stock, reduce heat, and simmer for 2 hours in a covered kettle. (If necessary, add more liquid.) Add potatoes, cabbage, and broccoli, and cook for another 15 minutes. Season to taste. Purée soup in a food processor, or mash the beans and vegetables, before serving.

SERVES 6

o o o

Lentil Soup

1 cup lentils, washed
4 cups water
4 tbsp. butter, margarine, or
  safflower oil
1 large potato, peeled and
  diced

3 stalks celery, sliced thin
2 carrots, scrubbed and
  sliced thin

Cook lentils (see page 148) in water until almost tender, about 30 minutes. Heat butter, margarine, or oil in a frying pan and in it gently sauté potato, celery, and carrots. (These vegetables can be added to lentils without sautéing first, if desired. Sautéing adds flavor.) Combine all vegetables with lentils, bring to a boil, reduce heat, and simmer for 10 minutes, or until vegetables are soft. For older children and adults, thyme, salt, and a vegetable, chicken, or beef bouillon cube may be added before simmering.

For infants and toddlers, purée or mash mixture to desired consistency.

SERVES 4

o o o

Split Pea Soup

1 onion, peeled and
  chopped
2 tbsp. olive oil
1 cup dried split peas,
  soaked overnight
4 cups water
½ tsp. thyme

1 bay leaf
1 large carrot, scrubbed and
  sliced
1 large potato, peeled and
  diced
1 tbsp. finely chopped
  parsley

(continued)

Sauté onion in oil until tender; set aside. In a large pot combine peas, water, thyme, and bay leaf. Bring to a boil and cook for 2 minutes. Let stand for 1 hour. Add onion, carrot, and potato, and simmer for 30 to 45 minutes. Remove bay leaf before serving and garnish with parsley.

SERVES 6

o o o

Syrian Lentil Soup

1 medium onion, peeled and chopped
1 tbsp. olive oil
1 cup lentils, washed
½ cup rice
6 cups lamb stock (or other meat stock) or water

10-oz. package frozen spinach, or bunch fresh spinach, washed and trimmed
1 tsp. salt
½ tsp. cumin
Juice of ½ lemon

Cook onion in oil in a large pot until soft. Add lentils, rice, and stock or water, and bring to a boil. Reduce heat and simmer gently for 1 hour. Add spinach, salt, and cumin, and cook for another 15 minutes. Stir in lemon juice before serving.

SERVES 6 TO 8

○ ○ ○

Vegetable Barley Soup

¼ cup barley
4 cups vegetable or chicken
   stock (see page 281 or
   page 280)
¼ onion, chopped
1 clove garlic, minced
1 tbsp. butter or margarine,
   or 2 tbsp. cooking oil

1 carrot, scrubbed and diced
1 small stalk celery, sliced
½ potato, scrubbed and
   diced
5 mushrooms, washed and
   sliced
½ tsp. thyme
2 tbsp. chopped parsley

Soak barley in cold water for 1 hour, drain, and combine in a large pot with 2 cups of the stock. Bring to a boil, reduce heat, and simmer for 45 minutes, covered, until barley is soft. In a skillet sauté onion and garlic in butter, margarine, or oil until tender. Add carrot, celery, potato, and mushrooms, and simmer for 10 minutes, stirring frequently. Add vegetables and thyme, plus remaining 2 cups stock, to barley. Simmer for 1 hour, stirring occasionally to prevent sticking. (Add more stock or other liquid if necessary to thin.) Add parsley just before serving.

SERVES 6

○ ○ ○

Yam Soup

1 tbsp. peanut or other
   vegetable oil
1 medium-size onion,
   peeled and chopped
2 tomatoes, peeled and
   chopped

½ lb. yams or sweet
   potatoes, peeled and
   cubed
1¼ cups vegetable or
   chicken stock (see page
   281 or page 280)
2 tbsp. chopped parsley

(continued)

Heat oil in a pot and sauté onion and chopped tomatoes in it until onion is tender. Add yams and stock, and bring to a boil. Reduce heat and simmer over low heat until yams are tender (about 30 minutes). Press mixture through a sieve, or blend or process, to achieve a purée. Return soup to pot to reheat. Garnish with parsley before serving.

SERVES 2

o o o

Homemade Chicken Soup

1 cup homemade chicken
   stock (see page 280)
1 tbsp. finely chopped
   cooked chicken
½ carrot, scrubbed and
   shredded
2 tbsp. pastina, or 3 tbsp.
   cooked rice

Bring stock to a boil in a saucepan, add all other ingredients, and continue to cook at a low boil for 5 minutes, or until carrot and pastina are done. Variations on this soup can be made by adding such vegetables as peas, beans, broccoli, spinach, squash (summer, banana, or acorn), or zucchini.

1 ADULT AND 1 CHILD SERVING

o o o

Chicken and Papaya Soup

1 chicken breast, boned and
  skinned
1 tbsp. vegetable oil
¼ onion, chopped
1 small clove garlic, minced
4 cups homemade chicken
  stock (see page 280) or
  water
1 tomato, peeled and
  chopped

½ unripe peeled papaya, cut
  into finger-width pieces
1 stalk lemon grass, washed,
  rubbed, and tied (4-inch
  strip of lemon peel can be
  substituted)
1 lb. fresh spinach, washed,
  stems removed
3 cups cooked rice

Cut chicken into 1-inch cubes and sauté in vegetable oil with
onion and garlic for 3 minutes, or until chicken is lightly
browned on all sides. Bring chicken stock or water to a boil
in a large pan. Add chicken mixture and chopped tomato. Reduce heat, cover, and simmer for 10 minutes, or until chicken
is tender. Add papaya and cook for 10 minutes more, adding
lemon grass after 5 minutes. The spinach should be added at
the last minute to preserve freshness and color. For each serving, place ½ cup cooked rice in a bowl and ladle soup over it.

SERVES 6

o o o

Chicken Soup with Speck
(Mini-dumplings)

Speck Batter (see below)   ½ carrot, scrubbed and
1 cup chicken stock (see   shredded
   page 280)   1 tbsp. finely chopped
                                      cooked chicken

Make batter. Bring stock to a boil in a saucepan. Dip a fork
into speck batter and shake batter off into boiling stock, using
about half the mixture. (Save remainder to use soon in another soup.) Add grated carrot and chopped chicken to soup,
and continue to cook at a low boil until carrots are tender.

SPECK BATTER

3 level tbsp. flour   1 egg, well beaten

Beat flour into egg until a smooth batter is formed. It should
be about the consistency of a pancake batter, not too thick
and not liquid.

1 ADULT AND 1 CHILD SERVING

o o o

Leftover Turkey Soup

Turkey carcass, stripped of   2 carrots, scrubbed
   all meat (reserve meat)   2 stalks celery, halved
1 medium-size onion,   Any leftover vegetables
   peeled and halved

Put turkey carcass in a large kettle and cover with water. Add onion, carrots, celery, and turkey meat. Bring to a boil, reduce heat, and simmer on very low heat for 3 hours. Remove bones from broth. Strain out vegetables through a sieve, and add leftover potatoes, peas, cauliflower, etc., to the soup. Add seasonings for adults.

SERVES 6 TO 8

o o o

Cholent
(Meat, Bean, and Vegetable Soup)

2 lbs. brisket of beef, trimmed of fat
2 tbsp. vegetable oil
1 onion, peeled and chopped
1 clove garlic, peeled and minced
1 cup dried lima beans, soaked overnight
½ cup barley
4 medium-size potatoes, peeled
4 carrots, scrubbed
2 turnips, peeled and halved
½ tbsp. paprika
1 tsp. salt
½ tsp. pepper
¼ tsp. each cinnamon and ground ginger (optional)
½ cup minced parsley

In a large Dutch oven, brown meat in oil together with chopped onion and garlic. Drain lima beans and add to meat, and add all other ingredients except parsley. Add enough boiling water to cover and bake in preheated 350° oven for 4 hours. To serve, break off pieces of meat from the brisket, cover with the soup, and garnish with parsley. Serve with challah bread (see page 246).

For infants and toddlers, purée or chop meat (and vegetables) to desired consistency.

SERVES 8

o o o

Pot-au-Feu

Plan to make this for a party or holiday.

5 lbs. beef bones
5 carrots, scrubbed
2 onions, peeled and
    quartered
2 leeks, white parts only,
    carefully washed
3 stalks celery, with tops,
    washed
1 tbsp. salt
Bouquet garni (2 bay leaves,
    4 sprigs parsley, 1 tbsp.
    thyme, 1 tbsp.
    peppercorns; tie in
    cheesecloth tightly and
    drop into pot)

¾ lb. lean beef, cubed
1 whole chicken, cut up
1 lb. Polish sausage
12 potatoes, peeled and
    halved
1 lb. carrots, scrubbed and
    cut into thirds
1 tsp. ground pepper
Bunch finely chopped
    parsley

The day before: Cook beef bones, carrots, onions, leeks, and celery in large pot of water with salt and the bouquet garni for 4 to 5 hours. Keep covered and constantly simmering. Let cool, then pour broth through colander lined with double layer of cheesecloth into another large pot. Discard all bones and vegetables. Refrigerate overnight.

The next day: Remove hard fat from broth, which will be like a gelatin, and return to heat, bringing slowly to a full boil. Add beef and chicken pieces and simmer for 1 hour. Finally, add sausage, potatoes, remaining pound of carrots, and ground pepper, and boil for 20 minutes, or until sausages and vegetables are cooked. Serve pot-au-feu sprinkled with plenty of chopped parsley. Accompany with crusty French bread.

This soup is perfect for all age groups. For under-two-year-olds, just purée or cut up finely some meat and vegetables. If desired, thyme, salt, or other seasonings may be added for adults.

SERVES 12 OR 16

o o o

Bean, Rice, and Vegetable Soup

1 onion, peeled and
 chopped
2 tbsp. olive oil
1 quart lamb or other meat
 stock
⅓ cup dried kidney beans,
 cooked (see page 146)
½ cup cooked or canned
 garbanzo beans (chick-
 peas)

½ cup lentils
⅓ cup raw long-grained rice
1 medium beet, cooked and
 cut into thin strips
1 cup cooked spinach,
 chopped
¼ cup lemon juice
Plain yogurt (optional)

Gently sauté onion in olive oil. In a large pot combine onion,
stock, kidney beans, garbanzo beans, lentils, and rice. Bring
to a boil, cover, and simmer for 1 hour. Add beet, spinach,
and lemon juice, and continue to simmer for 4 minutes before
serving to blend flavors. Top with yogurt, if desired.

SERVES 6

o o o

Black Bean Soup

½ cup dried black beans,
 soaked overnight
4 cups water
1 bay leaf
2 tbsp. vegetable oil
3 cloves garlic, peeled and
 sliced

1 onion, peeled and
 chopped
1 green or red sweet pepper,
 diced
½ tsp. cumin
1 tbsp. soy sauce
1 tbsp. chopped parsley

(continued)

Boil beans in water with bay leaf, reduce heat, and simmer for 20 minutes. Meanwhile, bring oil to medium heat in a skillet. Add garlic and onion and sauté until tender. Add pepper and cumin and sauté for 2 to 3 minutes more. Remove from pan, drain, add to beans when they have cooked 20 minutes, and simmer for another 20 minutes. Add soy sauce in the last minute or two of cooking, and garnish with parsley.

SERVES 4

o o o

White Bean and Cabbage Soup

4 oz. small dried white beans, soaked overnight
5 cups boiling water
1 bay leaf
8 oz. cooked ham, cubed
⅛ tsp. black pepper
¼ tsp. thyme

8 oz. cabbage, washed and shredded
½ onion, peeled and chopped
1 carrot, scrubbed and thinly sliced
1 turnip, peeled and chopped
¼ cup minced parsley
½ tsp. salt

Rinse beans well and place in a large pan. Cover with 5 cups boiling water, bring back to a boil, and cook for 2 minutes. Cover and let stand for 1 hour while preparing vegetables. Return beans to a boil, add bay leaf, ham, black pepper, and thyme, partially cover, and simmer for 1 hour until beans are tender. Remove bay leaf and add cabbage, onion, carrot, and turnip, and simmer for 1 more hour, still partially covered. Stir in parsley and salt before serving.

SERVES 4

o o o

Yellow Pea Soup with Vegetables and Sausage

1 cup dried yellow peas, soaked overnight
4 cups vegetable or chicken stock (see page 281 or page 280) or water
3 potatoes, peeled and diced

3 carrots, scrubbed and chopped
½ tsp. thyme
1 mild cooked sausage, chopped into 1-inch pieces (optional)

Bring peas to boil in stock or water, and cook until almost tender. Add all other ingredients, return to a boil, reduce heat, and simmer for 20 more minutes. Finely mash peas, potatoes and carrots, and chop optional sausage before serving to infants.

SERVES 6

o o o

Soup Dumplings

1 tbsp. butter or margarine
1 egg, beaten
3½ tbsp. all-purpose flour

Beat butter or margarine until soft, add egg, and mix well. Sift in flour and continue to mix until smooth batter is formed. Drop ¼ teaspoon of batter at a time into simmering soup or stew, and cook for 5 minutes.

BREADS

o o o

Challah

(Braided Egg Bread)

1 yeast cake or envelope dry
   yeast
½ cup lukewarm water
¼ lb. (1 stick) unsalted
   butter or margarine
½ cup warm milk
2 tsp. sugar
6 eggs, beaten

2 cups unbleached all-
   purpose flour
2 cups hard-wheat white-
   bread flour
½ tsp. salt
1 egg, beaten with 1 tsp.
   water
2 tbsp. sesame or poppy
   seeds

Lightly grease a large bowl and baking sheet and set aside.
Dissolve yeast in lukewarm water in a large glass or plastic
mixing bowl. Melt butter or margarine, add to warm milk,
then add sugar and stir over low heat until sugar is dissolved.
When temperature is approximately 100° add milk mixture to
yeast, then add beaten eggs. Sift in flours and salt, and mix
well until dough is formed. Turn out onto a lightly floured
board and knead until smooth and elastic (about 10 minutes).
Place dough in the greased bowl, turning to coat all sides, and
cover with a clean cloth. Set in a warm place and allow to rise
until double in volume, about 2 hours. Punch down dough,
knead briefly, and set aside for 10 minutes. Place dough on
lightly floured board and cut in half. Make 3 pieces out of
each half and roll each piece into a 12-inch-long rope. Lay 3

ropes beside each other and braid together loosely. Pinch both ends together to secure. Place loaf on a greased baking sheet. Repeat process with second half of the dough. Brush tops with beaten egg and sprinkle with seeds. Cover with a clean cloth and again allow to double in volume.

Bake loaves in preheated 350° oven for about 45 minutes, or until golden brown. Bread should sound hollow when tapped. Remove from baking sheet and cool on racks.

MAKES 2 LOAVES

o o o

Chapatis
(Indian Bread)

1 cup whole wheat flour
1 cup all-purpose flour
1 tsp. salt

2 tbsp. plus 1 tbsp. ghee
 (clarified butter)
¾ cup hot (not boiling)
 water from faucet

Put dry ingredients into a deep bowl, add 2 tbsp. ghee, and mix well with fingers. Add water with one hand while continuing to mix with the other. When dough becomes pliable and forms a smooth ball, stop adding water. Knead dough until it is very elastic. With pastry brush, cover dough with a thin film of ghee, and let stand while preparing to roll it out. Lightly flour a pastry board or other surface, then with hands, roll dough into a tube about 1½ inches in diameter. Cut pieces about the size of large eggs and form into round balls. Roll out with a rolling pin until each piece is approximately 6 inches in diameter and very thin. Preheat a griddle or skillet and cook chapatis for about 30 seconds on each side. Then, using tongs, hold each chapati over open flame until it puffs up. Remove immediately and brush with remaining ghee. Pile chapatis on top of one another under a clean cloth until all are cooked. Serve immediately.

MAKES 8 CHAPATIS

o o o

Corn Bread

1 egg
1 cup milk
1¼ cups unbleached white
    flour
¾ cup whole-grain cornmeal

2 tbsp. sugar
5 tsp. baking powder
¼ tsp. salt
2 tbsp. melted butter or
    margarine

Beat egg and mix with milk. Sift in all dry ingredients, add melted butter or margarine, and beat together until smooth. Butter a 9-inch pie dish and pour in batter. Bake in preheated 375° oven for 30 minutes, or until inserted toothpick comes out clean.

SERVES 6

○ ○ ○

Marion Cunningham's Health Bread*

2 envelopes active dry yeast
2 cups warm water, in all
4 tbsp. instant grain
  beverage (Postum)
⅓ cup dark molasses
⅓ cup cracked wheat
  (bulgur)

⅓ cup instant nonfat dry
  milk, or 1 cup whole milk
2 tsp. salt
½ cup toasted sunflower
  seeds
1 cup whole wheat flour
1 cup rye flour
3 to 4 cups all-purpose flour

Sprinkle yeast over ½ cup of warm water (115°) in a small bowl, stir, and let dissolve for 5 minutes. In a large bowl combine remaining water and all other ingredients, but *only 1 cup* of the all-purpose flour. Add yeast liquid and beat vigorously for 1 full minute, then add enough all-purpose flour to make a manageable dough. Turn dough out onto a lightly floured board, knead for 2 minutes, then let rise for 10 minutes. Add enough of remaining flour to dough so that it is not sticky, and continue kneading until it is smooth and elastic. Put dough in a large greased bowl, cover, and let rise until double in bulk in a warm, draft-free area. Turn dough out, punch down, and cut in half. Form each piece into a loaf and place in greased loaf pans. Cover pans lightly with clean towels and put in a warm spot to rise until dough reaches tops of pans. Make two diagonal slashes across the top of each loaf with a sharp knife. Bake in preheated 375° oven for 50 minutes. Remove loaves from pans and let cool on racks.

MAKES 2 LOAVES

o o o

Mexican Flour Tortillas

4 cups all-purpose flour
2 tsp. salt
½ cup vegetable shortening
1 cup lukewarm water

Sift flour and salt into a large mixing bowl. Add shortening
and with fingers mix until well blended. Add lukewarm water
and mix well. Turn dough out onto a lightly floured board
and knead 50 times. Divide dough into 12 equal pieces and
form each piece into a ball. Cover with a clean cloth and let
stand for 15 minutes. Roll out each ball into a round tortilla 8
inches in diameter. Cook on a moderately hot griddle, or in an
ungreased skillet, until golden brown in spots, turning once
without breaking the air bubbles.

MAKES 12 TORTILLAS

o o o

Norwegian Potato Bread

6 medium potatoes, peeled
    and cut up
¼ cup milk
¼ cup butter or margarine
2½ to 3 cups all-purpose
    flour

Boil potatoes until very soft. Drain (save water for soup or
stock). Mash potatoes thoroughly and whip in milk and butter
or margarine until light and fluffy. Cool in refrigerator. When
chilled, add half the flour and beat until smooth. Beat in

enough remaining flour to make a soft dough. Cut off pieces big enough to roll out into rounds ⅛ inch thick and 6 inches wide. Heat ungreased griddle until water drops bounce when dropped on it. Place potato-bread rounds on griddle and cook until brown spots appear. Turn and keep turning until bread is dry and lightly covered with brown spots. Cool and serve with butter and goat cheese.

The same recipe can be achieved with 1 cup leftover mashed potatoes, ½ cup all-purpose flour, and ¼ cup milk. Mix all ingredients into a smooth dough, adding extra flour if necessary to roll out easily. Then proceed as in original recipe.

MAKES APPROXIMATELY 1 DOZEN PIECES

○ ○ ○

Pita Bread
(Pocket Bread)

1 yeast cake or envelope dry
   yeast
1¼ cups warm water

3 cups wheat flour
1 tsp. salt
Vegetable oil as needed

Soak yeast in warm water (115°) for about 4 to 5 minutes. Sift in flour and salt and mix. Turn dough out onto a floured board and, moistening hands with oil, knead thoroughly, adding flour as needed. Divide dough into 6 pieces; knead each piece well and form into a ball. Roll each ball out on a floured board to make a 5-inch disk ¼ inch thick. Dredge pita disks lightly with flour, place on a clean towel, and cover with another towel. Leave for 45 minutes, or until breads are 1½ times larger than their original size. Place on an oiled cookie sheet and bake in preheated 500° oven for 3 to 5 minutes. Bread will puff up and will soften once it has cooled off.

MAKES 6 PIECES

o o o

Sesame-Seed Honey Bread

SPONGE MIXTURE

2½ tbsp. dry yeast
6 cups warm water

½ cup honey
4 cups whole-grain wheat
  flour

4 cups all-purpose flour
1 cup wheat germ
1 cup bran
1 cup sesame seeds

½ cup sesame oil
2½ tbsp. salt
2 egg yolks beaten with 2
  tbsp. water

In a nonmetallic bowl add ingredients for sponge mixture, mix, and let stand until mixture becomes foamy. Then beat 100 times with a wooden spoon. Cover with a damp cloth and set aside for 30 to 40 minutes. Punch down mixture, which will have risen, and add all other ingredients except egg yolks. Knead until smooth and elastic. Cover dough with damp cloth and let rise in a warm place until double in volume, about 30 minutes. Divide dough into 4 equal parts, shape, and place in greased loaf pans. Brush with egg yolk mixture, cover, and let rise for 15 to 20 minutes. Bake in preheated 350° oven for 20 to 30 minutes. Loaves are done if they sound hollow when tapped.

MAKES 4 LOAVES

o o o

Whole Wheat Bread

1 tbsp. dry yeast
2½ cups warm water
3 tbsp. honey

3 tbsp. sesame oil or other
   cooking oil
6 cups whole wheat flour
2 tsp. salt

Dissolve yeast in water (115°) and add honey and oil. Blend flour and salt, and sift into liquid mixture. Knead until smooth and elastic. Cover dough with a clean towel and allow to rise until double in size. Punch down dough, form into two loaves, and place in well-greased loaf pans. Let rise again to tops of pans and bake in preheated 350° oven for 30 minutes.

MAKES 2 LOAVES

o o o

Whole Wheat Crackers

1 cup whole wheat flour
¼ tsp. salt
¼ cup vegetable oil
3 to 4 tbsp. ice water

Sift flour and salt into oil in a bowl. Mix and add water, a little at a time. Dough should have texture of pie crust. Chill for 30 minutes or more. Roll out dough on a floured board until very thin. Using a pastry cutter, cut dough into squares, rectangles, or triangles. Place on an oiled cookie sheet and bake in preheated 350° oven for 10 to 15 minutes until crisp and lightly browned.

MAKES APPROXIMATELY 1 DOZEN CRACKERS

DESSERTS

Applesauce

2 sweet apples, peeled, cored, and quartered
⅓ cup water

Thinly slice apples and place in a small stainless-steel pan
with the water. Bring to a boil, reduce heat, and simmer, covered, for approximately 5 minutes, or until apples are tender.
Cool. Pour apples and liquid into a blender or food processor
and blend to desired consistency.

3 OR 4 CHILD SERVINGS

○ ○ ○

Baked Apples

1 red apple for each person, washed and cored
1 tbsp. seedless raisins each
1 pat of butter or margarine each

When coring apples, take care not to cut through bottom. Fill
center of each apple with raisins, cover with a pat of butter
or margarine, and stand apples in an ovenproof dish with
enough water to cover the bottom. Bake in preheated 350°
oven for 1 hour, or until apples are cooked through.

   For babies, mash apple and raisins after removing apple
skin.

SERVES 1

o o o

Apple Gel

2 cups apple juice
1 envelope unflavored gelatin

Put ½ cup apple juice in a bowl and sprinkle with gelatin. Let stand for 1 minute. Put remaining apple juice in a saucepan and bring to a boil, then add to the gelatin mixture. Stir until gelatin is completely dissolved. Pour into a mold or individual serving dishes and refrigerate until firm.

SERVES 4

o o o

Apple Mist

1 small sweet apple, peeled and cored
¼ cup apple juice
2 tbsp. cream

Slice apples, then cut slices in half. Put into a small saucepan with apple juice and simmer until apples are soft. Remove from heat and mash well. Add cream and mix with a wire whisk. Serve warm or cold.

1 CHILD SERVING

○ ○ ○

Homemade Apple Pie

PASTRY

1½ cups cake or all-purpose
 flour
½ tsp. baking powder
½ tsp. salt

⅓ to ½ cup shortening
 (butter or other fat)
¼ cup ice water
 (approximately)

FILLING

4 apples, peeled, cored, and
 sliced
3 tsp. butter or margarine

Cinnamon (optional)

Sift flour, baking powder, and salt into a large bowl. Cut shortening into flour with a knife until the size of peas. Then mix with hands, breaking up shortening very lightly until ingredients are of a crumblike consistency. Add ice water a little at a time until a firm dough is achieved. It is important not to add too much water. If mixture should become sticky, add a little more flour. Turn dough out onto a cold floured board or table, and divide into 2 pieces. With floured hands and rolling pin, roll out each piece until ½ inch thick. Fold in thirds and roll again. Repeat. Place dough in refrigerator for ½ hour, then roll out each piece until it is large enough to fit a 9-inch pie dish.

Grease pie dish, moisten edge of dish with water, and loosely lay one round of dough over dish. Gently press dough down into base and sides of dish and fill with apple slices. Dot with butter or margarine and sprinkle with cinnamon (if desired).

Roll out top crust, moisten edge of bottom crust with water, and cover pie with top layer. Trim off extra pastry, then pinch top and bottom layers of pastry together. Prick upper crust a couple of times with a fork. Place pie in preheated 450° oven for 12 minutes. Reduce heat to 350° and bake for 25 to 35 minutes more, or until crust is brown. (For a more golden and shiny crust, brush top with a mixture of milk and egg yolk before baking.)

SERVES 4 TO 6

○ ○ ○

Poached Apples

4 green (pippin) apples   2 tbsp. water
Juice of ½ lemon   Pinch ground cinnamon
⅔ cup fresh orange juice

Wash apples, cut into quarters, and remove cores and seeds. Slice segments thin and place in a lidded frying pan. Cover apples with all other ingredients. Cook over low heat, turning slices occasionally, until the apples are soft but not mushy. It is important to keep the apples covered to poach them (except when turning them).

SERVES 4

○ ○ ○

Apple Strawberry Parfaits

2 envelopes unflavored gelatin
3 cups apple juice
3 cups sliced strawberries

Sprinkle both envelopes of gelatin over 1½ cups cold apple juice and let stand for 1 minute. Heat remaining juice to boiling point and add to gelatin mixture, stirring until gelatin is

dissolved. Pour into an 8 × 8 × 2-inch baking dish and refrigerate until firm. Using a fork, break up gelatin into small pieces
and put a spoonful into each of 6 parfait glasses. Follow with
a layer of strawberries, another layer of gelatin, then more
strawberries, ending with a top layer of gelatin.

For a special treat or occasion, either whipped cream or ice
cream can be added as an extra layer or used as a topping.

SERVES 6

○ ○ ○

ABC (Apricots/Banana/Cream) Dessert

½ ripe banana, peeled
2 stewed apricots, puréed
1 tbsp. whipped cream

Mash banana to desired consistency, place in a small dish,
and top with puréed apricots. Serve with a dollop of whipped
cream.

1 CHILD SERVING

○ ○ ○

Cold Apricot Soup

1 lb. dried apricots
1 cup cream or half-and-half
4 tbsp. whipped cream (optional)

Cover apricots with warm water and soak for 1 hour. Blend apricots and soaking water in a food processor or blender until puréed. Strain mixture through a sieve, stir in cream, and chill. Serve with a dollop of whipped cream, if desired.

SERVES 4

o o o

Broiled Banana

½ large ripe, but firm, banana
1 tsp. unsalted butter or margarine, melted
1 tsp. lime or lemon juice

Place unpeeled banana under preheated broiler, about 5 inches from the flame, for 10 minutes, turning fruit once. Remove from heat with tongs, peel and mash banana, and mash again to desired consistency with butter or margarine and lime or lemon juice.

1 CHILD SERVING

o o o

Banana Coconut Pudding

2 eggs
1 ripe banana, peeled and
 mashed
¼ cup grated coconut

¼ cup milk, half-and-half, or
 light cream
½ tsp. vanilla extract

In mixing bowl, beat eggs. Add banana, coconut, milk, and vanilla extract, and stir ingredients until blended. Pour mixture into a small ovenproof casserole, then stand casserole in a larger pan almost filled with water. Place in preheated 350° oven and bake for 1 hour, or until set.

S ERVES 4

○ ○ ○

Banana Raita

1 tsp. ghee (clarified butter;
   see page 282)
⅛ tsp. ground cardamom
1 ripe banana
¼ cup yogurt

In a frying pan melt ghee with cardamom over medium heat. Mash banana well and mix with yogurt. When ghee is melted and bubbling gently, add banana to pan and stir vigorously. To serve this dish warm, just cook until heated through; to serve cold, mix the ingredients well, then remove from heat and chill.

1 ADULT AND 1 CHILD SERVING

○ ○ ○

Norwegian Birthday Cake

6 medium eggs
1 cup sugar
½ tsp. baking powder
1½ cups all-purpose flour

FILLING

2 packages frozen
  raspberries
Two 16-oz. cans raspberries

Two 8-oz. cartons cream,
  whipped
1 tsp. vanilla extract

Defrost frozen berries and strain all the raspberries, reserving juice. Beat eggs and sugar together with a hand mixer until very light. Mix baking powder with flour and sift into eggs and sugar, beat lightly until smooth, and pour mixture into a greased and floured round springform cake pan. Bake in preheated 350° oven for 45 minutes, or until a toothpick comes out clean when inserted. Place cake on a rack to cool, then turn out onto a plate. When cake is completely cool, cut in half horizontally, and soak both layers in all the reserved raspberry juice. (This part of the recipe may be made a day ahead. The cake should be covered and refrigerated until ready to finish.)

Cover bottom layer of cake with raspberries and then cover generously with whipped cream flavored with vanilla extract. Top with second layer and cover with remaining whipped cream. Decorate with fresh berries, flowers, candles, or as desired.

MAKES 10 OR 12 SERVINGS

o o o

Bread Pudding

2 cups stale bread, broken
  into pieces
2 cups milk
2 eggs, separated

3 tbsp. unsalted butter or
  margarine, melted
1 tsp. vanilla extract
⅓ cup raisins

Butter the sides and bottom of an ovenproof casserole and line with bread pieces. Pour milk over the bread to soften and let stand for 15 minutes. Meanwhile, beat together egg yolks, melted butter or margarine, and vanilla extract. Add mixture and raisins to bread and milk, and stir to mix. Beat egg whites until stiff and fold into mixture lightly. Preheat oven to 400°, set the casserole in a large pan half filled with water, and bake for 1 hour.

SERVES 4

o o o

Cottage Cheese Pudding

½ cup milk, or more if mixture needs thinning
2 cups small-curd cottage cheese

Juice and grated peel of ¼ lemon
¼ tsp. vanilla extract
½ tsp. ground cardamom

Put all ingredients in a blender or food processor, starting with the milk. Blend until smooth. Pour into individual dishes or bowl and refrigerate until set.

SERVES 4

o o o

Cranberry Cubes

3 cups cranberry juice
3 envelopes unflavored gelatin

Put 1½ cups cold cranberry juice in a large bowl and sprinkle with gelatin. Let stand for 1 minute. Meanwhile, heat remaining juice to boiling point. Add heated juice to gelatin mixture and stir until gelatin is completely dissolved. Pour into an 8-inch-square baking dish and chill until firm.

To serve, cut into 1-inch squares. This dessert is fun for children to decorate with fruits such as mandarin orange segments, slices of banana, pitted cherries or grapes, etc.

SERVES 6

o o o

Figs in Yogurt

6 fresh figs
¼ cup ground pistachios
   and almonds, well mixed
Orange juice for marinade

1 cup plain yogurt,
   preferably homemade (see
   page 149)
1 tbsp. honey
¼ tsp. vanilla extract

Wash figs, cut off tops, and carefully stuff 1 teaspoon ground nuts into each fig. Stand figs in a dish approximately 4 inches deep and cover with orange juice. Marinate for 45 minutes, then remove from juice with a slotted spoon. Mix ¼ cup orange juice marinade with yogurt, honey, and vanilla extract, and divide mixture among 6 small custard cups. Place a fig in each cup and chill until ready to serve.

SERVES 6

○ ○ ○

Fruit Compote

¼ lb. pitted dried prunes
¼ lb. pitted dried apricots
1 apple, peeled, cored, and
    diced
1 ripe pear, peeled, cored,
    and diced

Soak prunes and apricots overnight in a pan with enough water to cover. Using same water, bring fruit to a boil and add apple and pear. Bring back to a boil, reduce heat a little, and cook until fruit is soft and most of the liquid has been absorbed. Stir occasionally to prevent sticking. Serve warm or cold, with a little milk if desired. Purée compote for babies without teeth; mash to coarser texture for older children.

SERVES 4

○ ○ ○

Fruit Custard

2 egg yolks
½ cup puréed fruit (banana,
    plums, pears, peaches, or
    combination of any two)
¼ cup whole milk
¼ tsp. vanilla extract

Beat egg yolks well, add fruit, milk, and vanilla extract, and continue to beat until smooth. With a dot of butter, lightly grease 2 custard cups, pour mixture into cups, and bake in preheated 350° oven for 30 minutes, or until set.

1 ADULT AND 1 CHILD SERVING

○ ○ ○

Fresh Fruit Salad

1 small orange, peeled, seeded, and chopped (include juice)

1 apple, peeled, cored, and chopped

1 ripe banana, peeled and cut up

1 ripe pear, peeled, cored, and chopped

Put all ingredients in a bowl and mix well. For children, serve with a little cold milk, if desired.

SERVES 2

○ ○ ○

Grape Divine

1 envelope unflavored gelatin
2 cups grape juice

Sprinkle gelatin over ½ cup of the grape juice in a bowl and let stand for 1 minute. Bring remaining juice to a boil and add to the gelatin mixture, stirring until gelatin is dissolved. Refrigerate in the bowl until mixture is the consistency of unbeaten egg whites. Using electric mixer, beat at high speed until jelled mixture triples in volume (about 10 minutes). Chill until set.

SERVES 4

○ ○ ○

Kiwi Kwiki

1 kiwi fruit, peeled and sliced crosswise
½ ripe banana, peeled
1 tbsp. vanilla ice cream

Cut kiwi slices in half, and thinly slice banana. In a small dessert dish combine both fruits, saving two kiwi slices for decoration. Top with ice cream and finish with kiwi slices arranged like butterfly wings. An easy recipe to multiply to serve as many as you wish.

SERVES 1

○ ○ ○

Melon Berry Melba

¼ cup cranberry juice
¼ cup orange juice
1 cup fresh raspberries
2 cups cantaloupe balls

Freeze juices in ice cube tray, then lightly crush in blender. In 4 sherbet glasses divide up raspberries and cantaloupe balls, and drizzle crushed fruit ice over top. Serve immediately.

SERVES 4

○ ○ ○

Cold Melon Soup

¼ ripe cantaloupe, peeled and seeded
¼ cup orange juice
1 tbsp. plain yogurt

Cut cantaloupe into chunks and purée in a food processor. Add orange juice and yogurt, and blend until smooth. Chill well before serving. For a more elegant dessert, add small melon balls and/or a dollop of whipped cream and top with a sprig of mint.

1 ADULT AND 1 CHILD SERVING

○ ○ ○

Orange Cloud

½ cup orange juice
1 envelope unflavored
   gelatin
½ cup water
1 cup cold milk

Put orange juice in a bowl, sprinkle with gelatin, and let stand for 1 minute. Bring ½ cup water to a boil, pour over gelatin mixture, and stir until gelatin is completely dissolved. Slowly add cold milk and stir well. Pour into a mold or individual dessert cups and refrigerate until set.

4 CHILD SERVINGS

o o o

Norwegian Pancakes

2 eggs
1½ cups milk
¾ cup all-purpose flour

¼ tsp. cardamom
Vegetable oil for cooking
Blueberry jam for topping

Beat eggs in a bowl, add milk, and sift in flour and cardamom. Beat all ingredients except oil and jam lightly until a smooth thin batter is achieved. Heat 1 teaspoon oil in a small omelet or nonstick frying pan until almost smoking. Add just enough batter to coat bottom of pan, rotating pan to spread the batter very thin. Shake pan gently to prevent sticking, and when pancake is brown on one side, flip over with a spatula to cook the other side. (This should take only a few seconds.) Turn out onto a warm plate and serve immediately with jam.

For variations, fresh berries, peaches, pears, applesauce, sliced bananas, or ice cream for a special treat can be substituted.

MAKES 8 TO 12 PANCAKES, DEPENDING ON SIZE

o o o

Peachy Pudding

2 cups peach nectar
1 envelope unflavored gelatin
1 cup vanilla ice cream

Place ½ cup of the peach nectar in a large bowl and sprinkle with gelatin. Set aside while heating remaining nectar in a small saucepan. Combine gelatin mixture with heated nectar and stir until gelatin is dissolved. Chill until partially jelled, approximately 1 to 2 hours, then place in a blender with ice cream and blend until well mixed. Pour into an attractive dish and chill until firm.

SERVES 4

○ ○ ○

Pear Surprise

2 ripe sweet pears, peeled, halved, and cored
1 mandarin orange, peeled, seeded, and cut in pieces (or
   small can mandarin orange segments)
4 tbsp. plain yogurt or whipped cream

Trim a very small slice from the round side of each pear half, so it will sit level on a plate. Fill each hollow with 1 tablespoonful mandarin oranges, and cover with yogurt or whipped cream.

SERVES 4

○ ○ ○

Persimmon with Grapes

1 ripe persimmon
5 black grapes

Cut persimmon in half and remove center pith. Scoop out flesh with a spoon and cut into small pieces. Halve grapes and remove any seeds. Arrange in a small dish and serve with half-and-half, cream, or vanilla ice cream.

SERVES 1

o o o

Stewed Plums

12 ripe sweet plums
½ cup water
1 tsp. vanilla extract

Wash plums, cut in half, and remove pits. Put water in a saucepan, add plums, cover, and simmer until tender, approximately 15 minutes. Drain liquid from plums and save (for Plum Yum, next recipe). Purée plums in a food processor, blender, or food mill, adding vanilla extract. Cool a little before serving.

If plums are too tart for your baby, add a little mashed banana or papaya to the purée.

4 CHILD SERVINGS

o o o

Plum Yum

½ cup plum syrup (saved
   from stewed plums,
   preceding recipe)
¼ tsp. lemon juice

½ tsp. vanilla extract
1½ tsp. arrowroot, potato
   flour, or cornstarch

Mix syrup, lemon juice, and vanilla extract in a small saucepan and bring to a boil. In a cup mix arrowroot with a little water to a smooth thin consistency. Add slowly to boiling syrup, stirring constantly until syrup is clear and thickened. Remove from heat and let it cool and thicken. Serve with milk.

2 TO 3 CHILD SERVINGS

o o o

Raspberry Tarte

Pastry shell (following recipe)
¼ cup fresh raspberries
1 tbsp. vanilla-flavored whipped cream

Make pastry shell according to directions and let cool. Rinse raspberries and drain until dry, then fill shell. Top with whipped cream just before serving.

MAKES 1 TART

o o o

Pastry Shells

1 tbsp. corn oil
2 tsp. cold water
1½ tbsp. whole wheat flour
2 tbsp. all-purpose flour

Beat oil and water together with a fork, then sift in flours, and mix until a pliable dough is formed. Grease individual cupcake or pie tins 2½ inches in diameter. Divide dough into 4 pieces and press 1 piece into each tin, using thumb to make a thin, even crust. Bake in preheated 375° oven for 10 to 15 minutes until shells are a light golden brown. Cool, unmold, and fill with berries, applesauce, creamed chicken, etc.

MAKES 4 SHELLS

o o o

Rice Pudding

2 cups milk
2 eggs
1 tsp. vanilla extract
1 tbsp. vegetable oil
½ cup raisins

½ tsp. each cinnamon and
  grated lemon rind
  (optional)
2 cups cooked rice (white or
  brown)

With a fork, mix together milk, eggs, vanilla extract, and oil,
add raisins (plus cinnamon and lemon rind, if desired), and
combine mixture with rice in an ovenproof dish. Bake in preheated 300° oven until milk is absorbed but pudding is still
creamy (about 1 to 1½ hours). Stir occasionally during cooking.

SERVES 4

o o o

Rice and Apricot Pudding

½ cup cooked rice
½ cup cooked apricots with
  liquid
1 tsp. vanilla extract
Milk (optional)

Put rice, apricots, and vanilla in a food processor fitted with
steel blade, or in a blender, and process until puréed. If a
creamier consistency is desired, add a little milk while blending. Other fruits, such as cooked prunes, plums, or pineapple, can be substituted for the apricots.

2 OR 3 CHILD SERVINGS

o o o

Strawberry Banana Mold

1 bar white agar*
1½ cups water

1 package frozen
    strawberries, thawed and
    drained
1½ cups apple juice
1 banana, sliced

Break agar into pieces and soak in water in a saucepan for about 10 minutes. Purée half the strawberries in a blender with a little of the apple juice. Meanwhile, bring agar mixture to a boil. Add puréed strawberries, reduce heat, and simmer for 10 minutes, stirring frequently, then add remaining apple juice. Arrange remaining strawberries and sliced banana in the bottom of a mold lightly coated with vegetable oil, and gently pour puréed mixture over the fruit. Refrigerate until firm, usually 1 to 2 hours. Serve unmolded.

SERVES 4

*Agar is a gelatin derived from seaweed. It contains many minerals and is beneficial as a laxative. This tasteless jelling agent can be used in place of animal gelatin. As well as being available in bar form, agar also comes in flakes or granules. Basic proportions are 3½ cups liquid (water and/or fruit juice) to 2 tablespoons flakes or 1 tablespoon granules. For a softer jell, use 4 cups liquid.

o o o

Strawberry Fruit Soup

1 pint strawberries, washed
    and hulled
4 tbsp. lemon juice
2 tbsp. sugar, dissolved in a
    little hot water

2 cups plain yogurt (see
    page 149 for homemade)

(continued)

Blend strawberries, lemon juice, and sugar in a food processor or blender until smooth. Pour into a bowl and stir in yogurt. Serve chilled.

SERVES 4

○ ○ ○

Summer Delight

½ cup cubed ripe melon or watermelon
½ cup cubed fresh or canned pineapple
½ cup diced pear
½ cup diced apple
¼ cup orange juice

Combine all ingredients in a bowl and toss. Chill for at least 1 hour before serving.

SERVES 4

○ ○ ○

Tropical Treat

1 mango, peeled and pitted
¼ cup cream, whipped

Cut mango into small pieces and press through a sieve or food grinder. Gently fold in whipped cream and serve immediately.

1 ADULT AND 1 CHILD SERVING

o o o

Yogurt Ambrosia

½ ripe banana
3 tbsp. chopped fresh
  papaya
2 tbsp. plain yogurt (see
  page 149 for homemade)
5 drops lemon juice

Finely chop or mash banana together with the papaya and fold into yogurt. Add lemon juice and blend well.

1 CHILD SERVING

FRUIT AND MILK DRINKS

Apricot Avocado Zest

12-oz. can apricot nectar
½ cup milk
1 small ripe avocado, peeled, pitted, and cut in chunks

Combine all ingredients in a blender and process until smooth.

SERVES 2

○ ○ ○

Apricot Breakfast Shake

1 cup apricot nectar
1 cup plain yogurt
1 ripe banana, peeled and
    cut in chunks
3 ice cubes, cracked

Combine all ingredients in a blender and process until smooth and fluffy.

SERVES 2

○ ○ ○

Banana Butter Delight

½ ripe banana
2 tbsp. peanut butter
½ cup milk
4 ice cubes

Put all ingredients in a blender and process 1 minute, or until smooth.

1 CHILD SERVING

○ ○ ○

Banana Strawberry Smoothie

1 ripe banana, peeled and cut in chunks
1 cup strawberries, washed and hulled
1 cup ice-cold milk

Combine all ingredients in a blender, process until smooth, and serve.

SERVES 2

○ ○ ○

Buttermilk Fruit Shake

1 cup buttermilk
4 oz. frozen berries or orange juice

Combine all ingredients in a blender and process until smooth and frothy.

2 CHILD SERVINGS

○ ○ ○

Hawaiian Chiffon

4 cups pineapple juice
1 ripe banana, peeled and cut in chunks
Large handful ground almonds

Process well in a blender and serve immediately.

SERVES 4

○ ○ ○

Minty Treat

4 cups orange juice, well chilled
2 ripe bananas, peeled and cut in chunks
½ tsp. dried mint leaves

Place all ingredients in a blender and process well. Serve immediately.

SERVES 4

○ ○ ○

Orange Milk Whip

½ cup milk
½ cup orange juice

Mix in a blender or food processor for 10 seconds. Serve immediately.

1 CHILD SERVING

○ ○ ○

Papaya Shake

1 papaya, peeled, pitted, and cut in half
1 pint orange sherbet
2 cups milk

Put all ingredients into a blender and process until smooth and frothy.

SERVES 4

○ ○ ○

Raspberry Tofu Smoothie

½ pint raspberries (or other berries), rinsed
8 oz. tofu
3 ripe bananas, peeled and cut in chunks

Process in a blender until smooth and serve immediately.

SERVES 3 TO 4

○ ○ ○

Strawberry Heaven

1 cup plain yogurt
6 strawberries, washed and
  hulled
½ ripe banana
4 ice cubes

Combine ingredients in a blender and process until smooth.

2 CHILD SERVINGS

o o o

Tropical Cooler

¼ cup dried apricots
½ cup warm water
1 medium-ripe banana

1 mango, peeled and pitted
2 tsp. lemon juice
12 ice cubes, cracked

Soak apricots in warm water for 10 minutes, then place in a blender with water and add banana, mango, and lemon juice. Cover and process until smooth. Remove center of blender cover and gradually add cracked ice, blending at high speed. Continue to blend for 2 minutes until drink is smooth.

SERVES 4

STOCKS AND SAUCES

Chicken Stock or Broth

Carcass and leftover meat
    from roast chicken
2 stalks celery, washed and
    halved
2 carrots, scrubbed and cut
    into thirds

1 onion, peeled and
    quartered
1 bay leaf
1 tsp. salt
Water to cover

Place all ingredients in a large pot and bring to a boil. Reduce heat and cook at a low simmer for approximately 2 hours. When cool enough, strain broth, saving liquid and chicken meat, and discard everything else.

○ ○ ○

Fish Broth

1½ quarts cold water
2 lb. fish (can include
   scraps) cut into
   3 × 3-inch pieces
1 bay leaf
1 tsp. whole black
   peppercorns

1 leek, cut lengthwise and
   rinsed well
1 carrot, scrubbed
2 celery stalks, washed and
   halved

In a large saucepan, combine water, fish, and spices. Bring to a boil slowly over a low heat. Keep boiling for 15 minutes, removing scum as it appears with a large spoon. Add vegetables, cover the pan, reduce heat, and simmer for 25 minutes. Strain liquid through a sieve, and discard the fish and vegetables.

○ ○ ○

Vegetable Soup or Stock

2 large potatoes, scrubbed
   and cubed
1 cup shredded carrots
1 cup chopped celery
   (include leaves)
1 cup beet or turnip tops,
   parsley, or other leafy
   vegetable, chopped

1 onion, peeled and
   quartered
1 clove garlic, peeled
1 bay leaf
1 tsp. dried herbs (mixed, or
   as desired)
1½ quarts cold water

Put all ingredients in a large pot, bring to a boil, reduce heat, and simmer for 30 minutes. To serve as soup, remove bay leaf and purée briefly in batches in a blender. Serve warm. To serve as a clear broth or stock, strain out chopped vegetables through a sieve or cheesecloth. If not used immediately, store in refrigerator and reheat before using.

○ ○ ○

Fresh Herb Sauce

2 tbsp. cold water
3 tbsp. lemon juice
2 tbsp. fish broth (page 281)
   (optional)
Dash white pepper

½ cup hot (170°) melted
   unsalted butter or
   margarine
2 tsp. fresh tarragon, basil,
   dill, or chives, minced

In a small enamel saucepan put water, lemon juice, fish broth (if desired), and pepper, and bring to a boil. Pour into a food processor or blender and, with machine running, pour in hot melted butter or margarine a little at a time, but take no more than 20 seconds. Process for 5 seconds and add minced herb of your choice. Process 5 seconds more and serve.

MAKES 4 SERVINGS

○ ○ ○

Ghee
(Clarified Butter)

Ghee is butter that has had all its milk solids removed. It is used in many recipes from India and neighboring countries.

Melt 1 pound of butter in a heavy 1-quart saucepan over medium-low heat. The butter should bubble and foam, but do not let it burn. Skim off foam from top and discard. Continue to heat butter over low heat until it foams again. Skim off foam again, and repeat until all foam disappears and the butter is a clear yellow liquid. Remove from heat and let cool for 5 minutes. Strain into a glass container through cheesecloth or a fine sieve; stop when white sediment in the liquid comes to the surface.

If the ghee is absolutely pure, it can be stored for long periods of time without refrigeration. It will become solid if stored in the refrigerator, but can be liquefied by heating over a low flame.

o o o

Marinara Sauce

1 clove garlic, peeled
¼ cup olive oil
2-lb. can tomatoes

1 tsp. salt
½ tsp. oregano
1 tsp. chopped parsley

Gently sauté garlic in heated oil for a few minutes. Meanwhile, purée tomatoes in a blender or food processor and add to oil with all other ingredients, removing garlic clove if desired. Cook slowly for 20 minutes, stirring occasionally. May be made ahead and frozen for later use.

o o o

Tomato Sauce

3 tbsp. olive oil
3 cloves garlic, peeled and
    lightly crushed
1 large onion, peeled and
    chopped
28-oz. can tomatoes

28-oz. can tomato purée
Two 6-oz. cans tomato paste
1 tbsp. each oregano and
    basil, crushed
1 tsp. salt

(continued)

Heat oil in a skillet, add garlic and onion, and sauté until onion is golden. Chop tomatoes for a few seconds in a food
processor, and add to onion and garlic with all remaining ingredients. Stir well, bring to a boil, then reduce heat and simmer for 15 to 20 minutes. Cooked ground meat and/or sliced
sautéed mushrooms may be added, if desired.

This sauce freezes well and can be kept in sealed containers
for use as needed.

o o o

White Sauce

1½ tbsp. butter or margarine
1½ tbsp. all-purpose flour
1 cup liquid (equal parts broth and milk, or 1 cup milk, or 1
    cup chicken or vegetable broth)

In a heavy-bottomed saucepan (do not use aluminum), melt
butter or margarine over *low heat*. Blend in flour a little at a
time, stirring constantly with a wooden spoon until butter and
flour bubble. Cook for 2 minutes, still stirring, until mixture
is smooth. Remove from heat and set aside for a minute until
bubbling has stopped. Add liquid and beat vigorously with a
wire whip until sauce is completely blended and without
lumps. Return to moderate heat and stir with whip until sauce
comes to a boil. Simmer for 1 minute and cover until ready to
serve.

For thinner sauce, use 1 tablespoon each flour and butter
or margarine, and 1 cup liquid.

For thicker sauce, use 2 tablespoons each flour and butter
or margarine, and 1 cup liquid.

This basic sauce may be used in many ways and is especially
good with grated Cheddar cheese added, or sautéed sliced
mushrooms. Serve over fish, chicken, eggs, and vegetables.

o o o

Tahini Dressing

½ cup tahini*   2 tbsp. olive oil
½ cup lemon juice   Dash pepper
1 clove garlic, minced   Salt (optional)
2 tbsp. minced fresh parsley

Place all ingredients in a blender or food processor and process until smooth. If necessary, add a little water to thin to desired consistency.

*Tahini is sesame-seed paste, available in health-food or Middle Eastern grocery stores.

Microwave Cooking

MICROWAVE ovens are used in more than three quarters of all American homes. For busy parents, microwave cooking can be a fast, convenient, and healthy way to prepare meals for babies and toddlers—as well as everyone else in the family. Flavor, texture, and color are preserved, extra fat and salt are unnecessary, and, with shorter cooking times and little additional water added to most recipes, food retains more vitamins and minerals than with conventional cooking. However, to achieve optimum and safest results from your microwave oven, it is important to know its limits and dangers as well as its advantages.

For successful use of your oven, it is essential to know the wattage (power output). If you cannot find this information from your owner's manual, the oven itself, or the manufacturer, the following simple test will gauge your microwave output. Fill a glass measuring cup with exactly one cup of cold water; checking the time, microwave on high, uncovered, until the water begins to boil. Your wattage is:

> 600 to 700 if boiling takes less than 3 minutes;
> 500 to 600 if boiling takes from 3 to 4 minutes;
> 500 watts or less if boiling takes more than 4 minutes.

This information is important to establish the length of time it takes to cook, reheat, or defrost foods.

Most available microwave recipes, including those in *The Baby Cookbook Revised Edition*, are prepared in 700-watt ovens. Should you need to convert cooking times to suit your microwave wattage, use the following table:

EASY OVEN CONVERSION TABLE	
500-watt ovens	Add 40 seconds for each minute of cooking time.
600-watt ovens	Add 20 seconds for each minute of cooking time.
650-watt ovens	No adjustment needed.

Pointers for Safe Microwave Cooking
- Defrost meats and fish in the refrigerator overnight to remove ice crystals before cooking.
- Never refreeze foods that have been defrosted.
- Wrap or cover food to trap steam.
- Rotate foods during cooking (a carousel is a good investment if your microwave oven does not have one).
- Check internal temperatures in several spots after removing from oven. Temperatures for beef, pork, veal, and lamb should register between 160° and 170°F (77°C); and for poultry, 185°F (85°C).
- Observe standing time, as shown in directions.
- Cook all stuffing separately.
- Debone roasts before cooking.
- Use tempered glass for fatty foods.

DANGERS AND POTENTIAL PROBLEMS

Thorough cooking of meat, poultry, and fish is vital to prevent food-borne illnesses. A large percentage of marketed raw chicken, for example, is contaminated with the salmonella bacteria, a frequent cause of food poisoning. While conventional cooking usually destroys disease-causing microbes (bacteria), microwave cooking can pose potential problems if foods are unevenly cooked or heated, or do not get cooked thoroughly. (Of particular concern in this regard are roasts weighing more than two pounds, and stuffed chickens or turkeys.)

Uneven heating may also cause problems, including burns, when cooking or heating baby food. For safety's sake, always:

- stir food to distribute heat evenly;
- test food yourself before offering it to your baby;
- transfer food to a serving plate or bowl, especially if your toddler feeds himself.

Baby bottles should never be heated in the microwave oven. A bottle may feel cool to the touch on the outside, but the fluid inside may be extremely hot. Reports from hospital emergency rooms nationwide show an increase in mouth burns in infants and toddlers who were given bottles straight from a microwave oven.

Some prepackaged microwaveable foods include browning/crisping inserts known as heat susceptors. These are used extensively with such foods as French fries, fish sticks, pizza, waffles, and other breakfast products. Microwave-oven temperatures can reach as high as 500°F with some products and could potentially cause harmful chemicals in the packaging to leach into foods. Should you have reason to use heat susceptors for browning, do not microwave foods any longer than is recommended on the heating directions, do not reuse heat susceptors, and do not eat anything from a package that has become extremely browned or charred.

Also of concern are prepackaged food trays that may be used in conventional or microwave ovens. If heated to temperatures from 350° to 400°F, these too may cause transmission of toxic chemicals from the packaging to the food.

Research is ongoing on the possibility of toxic substances migrating from plastic into foods. Although no final conclusions have been reached, studies have shown that some transmission of toxins does occur, encouraging judicious use of plastics in cooking until more is known.

Until enough research is conducted to give us more information about these potential hazards, it is wise to exercise caution and common sense when heating or cooking with a microwave oven.

MICROWAVE COOKWARE

Generally, lead-free glass or ceramics are the best options for microwave cooking, although not all glass or ceramics are microwave-safe. A quick test can be made to clarify this, as follows:

> Place container to be tested in the microwave with another container of water and microwave for one minute. Remove immediately. If the empty container is very warm or hot, it is unsafe for the microwave. If the container is lukewarm, it is safe for reheating. If the container is cool, it is safe for cooking.

Most paper plates, towels, and bowls are safe to use in a microwave oven, but never use recycled paper, which may contain metal flecks and could spark, causing a fire. Also avoid using colored or patterned paper goods, which could "bleed" into food. Plain white paper towels are a good standby to absorb excessive liquids from certain foods, especially fatty meats.

Plastic containers, lids, and wraps should not be used in the microwave unless specifically labeled "Microwave Safe" or "For Microwave Use." Do not use margarine tubs or other reusable plastic containers in your microwave.

Do not use metal in your microwave, including metal-trimmed dishes and twist ties or clips from the ends of packages. (Solid blue or orange-red glazed ceramics are sometimes metal-based and should be avoided, if possible.) Metal blocks microwaves, preventing food from cooking, and can also cause a flash of light, which may damage your oven.

In spite of these necessary precautions, with care and proper use, your microwave oven can provide delicious and nutritious dishes, often in a fraction of the time required for conventional cooking.

FISH

In general, fresh or thawed fish fillets, covered and steam-cooked in the microwave oven, become perfectly moist and tender. As they take so little time to cook (see table page 292), and do not reheat well, prepare vegetables and other side dishes first.

FRESH VEGETABLE COOKING TABLE (Based on cooking in a 700-watt oven)				
Vegetable	*Preparation*	*Amount*	*Cooking Time*	*Standing Time*
Asparagus	1½" pieces	1 lb.	6–7 min.	3 min.
Green/wax beans	1½" pieces	1 lb.	8–10 min.	—
Beets	Sliced	1½–2 lbs.	14–16½ min.	5 min.
Broccoli	Spears	1 lb.	7½–10 min.	—
Brussels sprouts	Whole	10-oz. tub	7–9 min.	3 min.
Cabbage	Chopped	1 lb.	8–10 min.	5 min.
Cabbage	Wedges	1 lb.	9–11½ min.	5 min.
Carrots	Sliced	1 lb.	8–10 min.	5 min.
Cauliflower	Florets	1 med. head	8–10 min.	3 min.
Cauliflower	Whole	1 med. head	13–19 min.	5 min.
Celery	½" slices	1 lb.	13–15 min.	5 min.
Corn on cob	Husk on	4 ears	12–15 min.	5 min.
Eggplant	Cubed	1 lb.	9–10 min.	3 min.
Eggplant	Whole, pierced	1–1¼ lbs.	6–10 min.	5 min.
Leeks	Whole, ends	1 lb.	12–13 min.	5 min.
Mushrooms	Sliced	1 lb.	5–7½ min.	3 min.
Onions	Whole, peeled	8–10 small	12–18 min.	5 min.
Peas	Shelled	1 lb.	6–9 min.	—
Parsnips	Cubed	1 lb.	10–13 min.	5 min.
Potatoes, sweet	Whole	8 (6 oz. each)	20–22 min.	5 min.
Potatoes, white	Whole	4 (6 oz. each)	12–15 min.	5 min.
Rutabaga	Cubed	4 cups	15–17 min.	5 min.
Spinach	Whole leaf	1 lb.	6–7½ min.	—
Squash	Sliced	1 lb.	9–10 min.	5 min.
Squash, summer	Cubed	1 lb.	9–10 min.	3 min.
Squash, winter	Halved, membrane removed, cooked facedown	1 lb.	13–15 min.	5 min.
Turnips	Cubed	4 cups	13–15 min.	3 min.
Zucchini	Sliced	1 lb.	9–10 min.	3 min.

FISH AND SHELLFISH COOKING TABLE				
Fish	Amount	Power Level	Cooking Time	Standing Time
Med. fish fillets	1 pound	High	4–6½ min.	3–5 min.
Med. fish fillets	2 pounds	High	7–10½ min.	3–5 min.
½"-thick fish fillet	4 ounces	High	1–3 min.	1 min.
3/4"-thick fish fillet	6 ounces	High	3–4 min.	1 min.
Fish steaks	1 pound	High	4–6½ min.	5–6 min.
Whole fish	1½–2 lbs.	High	7–10 min.	3–5 min.
Scallops	1 pound	High	5½–6½ min.	1–2 min.
Shrimp	1 pound	High	5 min.	1–2 min.

CHICKEN

This most versatile food is now available in markets conveniently packaged as chicken tenders or tender cuts. These small cutlets are quick to cook, easy to prepare, and use only breast meat, with no skin or bone. If you cannot find them, whole, skinless, boneless chicken breasts may be cut into 5 × 1-inch strips with similar results. In recipes calling for chicken tenders, canned chicken may also be substituted, but should be washed carefully to remove most of the high level of salt it contains (around 250 mg. per 2½-oz. serving).

Chicken tenders work well in a large variety of recipes. To prepare them very simply for a young child, cut into small pieces, removing tendon, arrange on a plate, cover, and microwave on high for 40 seconds. Slightly large pieces make an excellent finger food for toddlers. For infants, purée the cooked chicken with broth, water or milk.

DEFROSTING TABLE				
	Amount	*Power Level*	*Defrost Time*	*Standing Time*
Fish fillets	1 lb.	Defrost	5–7 min.	5–10 min.
Fish steaks	1 lb.	Defrost	5–7 min.	5–10 min.
Whole fish	1½–2 lbs.	Defrost	4–5 min.	5–10 min.
Whole chicken	3–4 lbs.	Defrost	24–28 min.	20 min.
Chicken parts	2½–3 lbs.	Defrost	12–15 min.	15 min.
Chicken breasts (with bone)	2–3 lbs.	Defrost	8–12 min.	20 min.
Chicken breasts (boneless)	1 lb.	Defrost	5–7 min.	5–10 min.
Chicken drumsticks	1 lb.	Defrost	7–8 min.	10 min.
Chicken thighs	1 lb.	Defrost	7–8 min.	10 min.
Chicken wings	1½ lbs.	Defrost	6–10 min.	10 min.
Turkey breast (with bone)	4–5 lbs.	Cook, then Defrost	4½ min. then 10–15 min.	20 min.
Turkey parts	2–3 lbs.	Defrost	12–15 min.	15 min.
Ground beef	1 lb.	Defrost	8–10 min.	10 min.
Cubed steak	1 lb.	Defrost	7–8 min.	10 min.
Flank steak	1½ lbs.	Defrost	9–10 min.	10 min.
Round steak	2 lbs.	Defrost	10–14 min.	10 min.
Sirloin steak	2 lbs.	Defrost	10–12 min.	10 min.

To prevent spread of bacteria, wash surfaces, utensils, and hands with hot, soapy water after handling chicken.

Place all frozen foods on a dish to catch juices. Defrost only as long as necessary, separating pieces as soon as possible. To avoid overdefrosting, check at minimum time, remove as soon as possible, and observe standing times.

INTRODUCTION TO MICROWAVE-COOKED BABY FOODS

We believe microwave cooking has revolutionized the concept of homemade baby food. Because foods cook so quickly in the microwave oven, the taste, color, and texture are maintained. Additionally, no seasonings, butter, or sauces are necessary to enhance the natural flavors.

In less time than it would take to defrost frozen vegetables or meats, or to heat up commercial baby foods, you can microwave a large variety of fresh, healthy, and delicious foods for your baby and family. An added bonus: no extra pans to clean up!

Although you will want to use freshly prepared vegetables for most meals, the microwave is a quick and convenient way to reheat leftover main meals, rice, and potatoes.

To avoid mouth burns, it is important that all heated baby foods be stirred and tested for coolness before serving. This cannot be too strongly emphasized.

For health's sake, keep your microwave oven and carousel spotless. If you do not have a 700-watt microwave, use the conversion table (page 287), and enjoy this excellent method of preparing your baby's meals on a regular basis.

BREAKFASTS

Breakfast is the most important meal of the day, but working parents are often hard-pressed for time to cook a substantial meal in the mornings. Studies continue to show that a nutritious breakfast can enhance academic performance, may play a role in keeping cholesterol values lower (so long as breakfast doesn't consist of eggs, bacon, hash browns, and Danish every day), and that people who eat healthy breakfasts run lower blood-cholesterol levels on average than those who skip breakfast. Another study shows that breakfast eaters tend to be leaner, which is important to keep in mind in view of the increasing trend toward obesity in children.

Easy and healthy breakfasts can be prepared quickly in the microwave oven, and can usually be served in the bowl they are cooked in, leaving no pots or pans to be washed! Cereals, eggs, fruits, and vegetables, with a variety of combinations, can be microwaved, as well as alternated with yogurt, wheat waffles, muffins, and toast, and juices or smothies (which children love). You can find recipes for delicious fruit and milk drinks on pages 275–280.

Hot cereals microwave very well and can be adapted to growing children's needs by gradually thickening the consistency with more cereal. Start with rice cereal, progress to oatmeal, then barley. From eight to twelve months of age, corn and wheat cereals (cream of wheat, millet, cornmeal, and buckwheat) may be added.

Baby Cereal: Mix 4 tbsp. cereal with ¼ to ½ cup liquid (use breast milk, formula, water, or juice, depending on the liquids your baby is taking) in a 2-cup glass bowl. Microwave cereal, uncovered, on medium for 15 to 30 seconds. Stir well and taste for coolness in several places before serving.

o o o

Apple, Orange, and Pear with Yogurt

2 tbsp. butter or margarine
1 tsp. vanilla extract
1 tbsp. brown sugar
  (optional)
1 medium apple, cored and
  cut into ⅛-inch slices

1 medium pear, cored and
  cut into ⅛-inch slices
1 medium seedless orange,
  peeled and sliced
6 tbsp. plain yogurt

(continued)

Melt butter or margarine in small glass bowl covered with plate on medium for 1 minute. Add vanilla extract, and brown sugar if desired.

On three small microwave-safe plates, arrange slices of fruit, sprinkle with melted-butter mixture, and cook on high for 3 minutes. Cool slightly. Top each serving with 2 tbsp. of plain yogurt. (This is a delicious breakfast, lunch, or dinner dessert.)

SERVES 3

○ ○ ○

Apricot and Prune Whip

⅓ cup water
5 dried apricots
5 pitted prunes

½ tsp. vanilla extract
¼ slice lemon (optional)
3 tbsp. plain yogurt

In 1-cup bowl, combine water, apricots, prunes, vanilla extract, and lemon (if desired). Cover with plate, and microwave on high for 3 minutes. Remove lemon if using. In food processor or blender, purée mixture with plain yogurt until smooth. (This is a wonderful topping for waffles, crackers, or toast.)

2 CHILD SERVINGS

○ ○ ○

Quick Cream of Wheat

2 tbsp. instant cream of wheat
½ cup milk
½ tsp. butter or margarine

In 2-cup bowl, mix cream of wheat with milk. Cook, uncovered, on high for 1 minute. Stir and cook for 30 seconds more. If a thicker consistency is desired, cook for another 30 seconds. Stir well, dot with butter or margarine, and serve with cold milk to taste.

Check carefully to ensure the cereal is not too hot for your child.

1 CHILD SERVING

○ ○ ○

Warm Grapefruit Crunch

1 grapefruit, halved, pitted,
   and sectioned
2 tbsp. brown sugar or
   honey (honey should not
   be served to children
   under age one)
4 tbsp. cottage cheese
2 tbsp. Grape-Nuts cereal

Put grapefruit halves into ½-cup microwave-safe bowls. Sprinkle brown sugar or honey over each half, and microwave on high for 1 minute. (If only one half of the grapefruit is used, cook for 30 seconds.)

Remove from oven. Top each half with cottage cheese and Grape-Nuts.

SERVES 2

○ ○ ○

Grits

1 cup cold water
¼ cup hominy grits

Combine water and grits in 4-cup bowl, cover tightly with microwave-safe wrap, and cook on high for 5 minutes. Remove
bowl from oven with pot holders and remove wrap carefully
away from you. Stir cereal and serve.

For variation you may add 1 tsp. honey (honey should not
be served to children under age one) or maple syrup, or 1
tbsp. raisins, microwaved on high for 1 minute in water or
apple juice.

SERVES 2

○ ○ ○

Bibai's Yummy Muffins

¾ cup all-purpose flour
¼ cup quick-cooking rolled
    oats
½ tsp. baking powder
½ tsp. baking soda
⅛ tsp. ground cinnamon
¼ cup packed brown sugar

¼ cup raisins
1 egg
2 tbsp. vegetable oil
½ cup buttermilk
12–14 large paper cupcake
    cups

In 4-cup mixing bowl, combine first seven ingredients and mix
with fork. In 1-cup bowl, whisk egg, oil, and buttermilk together. Combine all ingredients until well blended.

Make double cups with cupcake cups, and divide mixture
equally among 6 or 7 forms. Place in an outer ring on microwave turntable. Cook on high for 2 to 2½ minutes. Remove

from oven, take muffins out of paper cups immediately, and cool on wire rack.

MAKES 6–7 MUFFINS

o o o

Oatmeal on the Run

¾ cup water
½ cup rolled oats

Place water and oats in 2-cup bowl and microwave on high, uncovered, for 2½ minutes. Stir and serve. (Cold milk may be added to taste.)

For variations, add 3 dried apricots, finely chopped with ¼ tsp. grated dried orange peel; 2 tbsp. raisins with ¼ tsp. grated dried lemon peel; or ¼ cup fresh sliced strawberries or peaches.

SERVES 1

o o o

Polenta Breakfast Scramble

Scant ¼ cup yellow
  cornmeal
1 egg, beaten
2 breakfast sausages,
  precooked and cut into
  small pieces

¼ cup Parmesan cheese
  (optional)
1 cup water
½ tsp. olive oil

Combine all ingredients in 4-cup glass bowl and mix well. Cover and cook on high for 3 minutes, stirring halfway through. Serve with cantaloupe.

SERVES 1

o o o

Scrambled Eggs

1 tbsp. butter or margarine   ½ cup grated cheese
2 tbsp. milk or water   (optional)
4 eggs, well beaten   1 tbsp. chopped chives
                                               (optional)

Add butter or margarine and milk or water to 4-cup bowl and
microwave on high for 45 seconds. Add eggs, whisk, and
cook, uncovered, on high for 1 to 1½ minutes. Fluff with fork,
cook for 1 more minute, and fluff again. Eggs should be
slightly moist. If still too liquid, cook for another 20 to 30 seconds until set. If desired, stir in grated cheese and/or chopped
chives.

SERVES 2

o o o

Egg Scramble for Child

1 tsp. butter or margarine
1 tbsp. milk
1 egg, well beaten

Add butter or margarine and milk to 1-cup bowl, cover with
plate, and cook on high for 30 seconds. Add egg and mix well
with fork. Microwave, uncovered, on high for 30 seconds, and
fluff with fork. If too moist, cook 5 to 10 seconds more.

   For variation, stir 1 tbsp. of plain yogurt, ricotta, or cottage
cheese into egg scramble.

1 CHILD SERVING

○ ○ ○

Egg Pastina

1 cup water
3 tbsp. pastina

Combine water and pastina in 4-cup glass bowl. Cook, uncovered, on high for 5 minutes. Let stand for 1 minute. Serve with a dot of butter or margarine and a little milk.

For variation, add 1 tbsp. raisins. First microwave them on high for 1 minute in ¼ cup of water or apple juice. You could also add sliced banana, strawberries, or kiwi fruit. Top with 1 tbsp. applesauce, or Apricot and Prune Whip (see recipe, page 296).

1 CHILD SERVING

○ ○ ○

Buòn Giorno Omelet
(A special, colorful omelet for breakfast or brunch)

4 slices bacon
1 tbsp. chopped onion
1 cup frozen hash brown
  potatoes
2 tbsp. each diced red and
  green bell pepper

4 eggs, beaten
3 tbsp. milk
⅓ cup grated mozzarella,
  Swiss, or Cheddar cheese

Cover bacon with plain paper towels, place in 4-cup casserole, and microwave on high for 3 to 4 minutes. Remove paper towels and any excess fat, break up bacon, and return to casserole along with onion, potatoes, and peppers. Cook 4 minutes on high, stirring once. In the meantime, whisk together eggs and milk. Combine with hash browns, onion, peppers, and bacon, and microwave on medium high for 4 minutes, or until eggs are set, stirring once. Cover with cheese and let stand until cheese melts. Serve immediately.

SERVES 2

o o o

Poached Egg

1 tbsp. water
¼ tsp. white vinegar
1 egg

Using a custard cup or a 4-oz. glass bowl, combine water and vinegar and microwave on high for 30 seconds. Crack egg into vinegar-water and prick yolk with fork. Cover with small plate and microwave on medium for 1 minute. Let stand for 1 minute, covered, drain, and serve.

SERVES 1

o o o

Egg with Refried Beans, Salsa, and Cheese

¼ cup refried beans (see
  pages 179–180) or canned
1 tbsp. mild salsa (or spicy,
  if preferred)

2 tbsp. jack, mozzarella or
  Cheddar cheese, grated
1 egg

Place beans in bottom of a ramekin or custard cup. Cover with salsa and cheese. Break egg over cheese, prick yolk with toothpick or fork. Cover with paper towel and microwave on medium high for 1 to 1½ minutes, or until egg white is set.

SERVES 1

o o o

Huevos Rancheros Presto

1 egg
1 tbsp. water
1 tortilla (corn or flour)
1 tsp. grated mozzarella
   cheese
1 tbsp. salsa (mild, or to
   taste)

In small glass bowl, whisk together egg and water. Microwave on high for 30 seconds. Place tortilla on plate, cover with egg, which will still be running. Cover with cheese and salsa. Microwave on high for 40 seconds, or until egg is set. Roll up tortilla and serve immediately with refried beans (canned or homemade).

SERVES 1

VEGETABLES

Potatoes, Sausage, and Egg Scramble*

1 tbsp. safflower oil
½ cup frozen hash brown
   potatoes
2 tbsp. milk
1 (frozen) fully cooked
   breakfast sausage

1 tsp. butter or margarine
1 tbsp. milk
1 egg

Pour oil onto small microwave-safe plate. Add frozen hash browns, cover, and microwave on high for 3 minutes. Remove, add 2 tbsp. milk, and mash with fork. Place frozen sausage on white paper towel or napkin, and cook on high for 30 seconds. In 1-cup capacity bowl, microwave 1 tbsp. butter or margarine and 1 tbsp. milk on high for 30 seconds. Add egg and whisk lightly with fork. Cook uncovered on high for 30 seconds, then fluff with fork. If still too liquid, cook for 10 seconds more, fluff again, and serve on warm plate with potatoes and sausage.

SERVES 1

*Hash brown potatoes do not brown or crisp well in the microwave oven, but they can quickly be turned into tasty mashed potatoes.

○ ○ ○

Beets

One 2-inch beet, greens removed, well washed
Water to cover

Prick skin of beet with fork, place in 1-cup glass bowl, cover
with water, and microwave on high for 3 to 4 minutes (a 1-
inch beet will take 2 minutes). Rinse under cold water and
peel. Can be puréed, mashed, or cut up for finger food (which
can be messy).

Beets mix well with cooked peas, carrots, green beans, potato, celery, sweet potato, spinach, zucchini, or other squash,
cauliflower, broccoli, apple, pear, cottage cheese, or yogurt.

1–2 CHILD SERVINGS

○ ○ ○

Carrots

2 tbsp. sliced carrot
2 tbsp. water or apple juice

Place 2 tbsp. of carrots in ½-cup glass bowl. Add 2 tbsp. water
or apple juice, cover, and microwave on high for 2 minutes.
Purée, mash, or serve as finger food, depending on child's
age. More liquid may be needed to purée carrots. (To double
the portion, double liquid and cooking time.)

Carrots mix well with yogurt, cottage cheese, cooked potato, yam, celery, spinach, green beans, beets, peas, zucchini,
broccoli, turnip, or rutabaga.

1 CHILD SERVING

○ ○ ○

Carrot with Pear

2 tbsp. sliced carrot
½ pear (or apple), peeled and cored
2 tbsp. water

Combine all ingredients in small glass bowl, and microwave on high for 3 minutes. Purée, mash, or serve as finger food.

1 CHILD SERVING

○ ○ ○

Dill Carrots Julienne

½ lb. carrots, well scrubbed
1 tbsp. butter or margarine
½ tsp. dill

Julienne (very thin sticks) carrots, then place in 2-cup bowl with butter or margarine and dill. Cover with plate and microwave on high for 6 minutes, or until tender. Stir and serve.

SERVES 3 TO 4

○ ○ ○

Cauliflower

One 2-inch caulifloweret, rinsed
1 tbsp. water

Place cauliloweret and water in small glass bowl, cover, and microwave on high for 1 minute. (To purée or mash, use 2 tbsp. water and cook for 2 minutes.)

1 CHILD SERVING

○ ○ ○

Cauliflower and Carrot

One 2-inch caulifloweret
2 tbsp. sliced carrot
4 tbsp. water

Combine all ingredients in ½-cup glass bowl, cover, and microwave on high for 3 minutes. Purée, mash, or serve as finger food, depending on child's age.

1 CHILD SERVING

o o o

Celery

2 tbsp. celery, washed and thinly sliced
1 tbsp. water

Combine celery and water in ½-cup glass bowl. Cover and microwave on high for 2 minutes.

Celery combines nicely with cooked carrot, beets, tomato, red pepper, yam, potato, apple, or pear.

1 CHILD SERVING

o o o

Celery with Red Pepper and Apple

1 tbsp. celery, washed and
   thinly sliced
1 tbsp. red pepper, washed
   and finely chopped
¼ apple, peeled and cored
1 tbsp. water

Combine all ingredients in ½-cup glass bowl. Cover and microwave on high for 1 minute.

1 CHILD SERVING

○ ○ ○

Green Beans

2 tbsp. green beans, washed and cut into ½-inch pieces
1 tsp. water

Combine green beans and water in ½-cup glass bowl. Cover
and microwave on high for 2 minutes. Additional liquid may
be added to purée or mash beans.

1 CHILD SERVING

○ ○ ○

Green Beans with Carrot and Apple

1 tbsp. green beans, washed
    and cut into ½-inch pieces
1 tbsp. thinly sliced
    scrubbed carrot
1 tbsp. water
¼ apple, peeled, cored, and
    cubed

Combine beans, carrot, and water in ½-cup glass bowl. Cover
and microwave on high for 2 minutes. Add apple and continue cooking for 30 seconds more.

1 CHILD SERVING

o o o

Green Beans with Red Pepper

1 tbsp. olive oil
2 large cloves garlic, peeled
  and minced
2 tbsp. sweet red pepper,
  chopped
1 cup green beans, cut into
  1-inch pieces

Place olive oil, garlic, and red pepper in 2-cup glass bowl and microwave, uncovered, on high for 1 minute. Add green beans, stir, and sprinkle with water. Continue to microwave on high for another 3½ to 4 minutes.

SERVES 2

o o o

Green Beans with Tomato

2 tbsp. green beans, washed and cut into ½-inch pieces
½ tomato, blanched and chopped (see page 148), or canned

Combine beans and tomato in ½-cup glass bowl, cover, and microwave on high for 2 minutes. Purée or mash, if necessary.
  For variation, a 2-inch caulifloweret may be used in place of tomato.

1 CHILD SERVING

○ ○ ○

Potatoes

1 medium or large baking potato, scrubbed

Prick potato with fork, and microwave on high for 6 minutes, or until soft. (Smaller potatoes will take less time, as will firmer potatoes for finger foods.) Scoop potato out of skin and mix with any of the following: cooked carrot, beets, broccoli, yam, cauliflower, peas, beans, spinach, turnip, rutabaga, apple, pear, cottage cheese, or yogurt. Add milk, broth, or juice, if needed.

1 ADULT AND 1 CHILD SERVING

○ ○ ○

20-Minute Baked Potatoes

4 medium baking potatoes, well scrubbed

Prick each potato twice with a fork, arrange evenly on microwave carousel, and cook on high for 10 minutes. While they are cooking, heat conventional oven to 400°F, transfer potatoes to top rack, and cook in conventional oven for another 7 to 10 minutes. This will make potato skins crisp and potato fluffy.

SERVES 4

○ ○ ○

Potatoes Au Gratin

2 tbsp. butter or margarine
½ cup grated Cheddar
   cheese
1½ tbsp. flour
2 tsp. chopped chives

½ tsp. dry mustard
⅛ tsp. pepper
1⅓ cups milk
2 medium potatoes, peeled
   and sliced ⅛-inch thick

Microwave butter or margarine in 8-cup glass bowl for 45 seconds, or until melted. Stir in cheese, flour, chives, mustard, pepper, and milk. Microwave on high for 5 minutes, or until thickened, stirring once. Arrange potato slices in a glass pie dish, pour over cheese-sauce mix, and cover with plate. Microwave on high for 10 minutes. (To brown the potatoes, dish may be popped under the grill of a conventional oven for 2 or 3 minutes, with a little extra grated cheese if desired.)

SERVES 3 TO 4

○ ○ ○

Thai Curried Potatoes and Peas (Mild)

1 tbsp. vegetable oil
1 clove garlic, peeled and
   crushed
1 tsp. curry powder
1 large potato, peeled and
   cubed

½ cup frozen peas
½ cup chicken broth
½ cup unsweetened coconut
   milk (canned)
2 tsp. Thai fish sauce
   (optional) (available in Far
   Eastern and specialty
   stores and occasionally in
   the Oriental section of the
   supermarket)

In 4-cup glass bowl, combine oil, garlic, and curry powder, and microwave on high for 1 minute. Add potato, peas, chicken broth, and coconut milk. Cover with plate and microwave for 10 minutes on high, or until potatoes are cooked. Add fish sauce, if desired, and stir.

SERVES 2

o o o

Rutabagas

¼ cup peeled and chopped rutabaga
4 tbsp. water

Combine rutabaga and water in 1-cup glass bowl. Cover and microwave on high for 4 minutes. Serve as a finger food. (For puréeing or mashing, cook for 2 to 3 minutes longer.)

Alternative method: Wash and prick skin of small rutabaga. Microwave whole on high for 5 minutes. Peel and cut up.

Rutabagas blend well with carrots, parsnips, turnips, peas, and green beans.

1 CHILD SERVING, CHOPPED

1 ADULT AND 1 CHILD SERVING, WHOLE

o o o

Sweet Potato or Yam

1 medium sweet potato or yam, scrubbed

Prick skin 2 or 3 times, and microwave on high for 7 minutes, or until potato feels soft.

For variation, peel and core half of a ripe apple or pear, and cut up. Microwave in small bowl for 30 seconds. Mix with sweet potato or yam.

Sweet potatoes and yams combine well with cooked carrots, apples, pears, cottage cheese, or yogurt.

1 ADULT AND 1 CHILD SERVING

For 1 child serving:

Cut a 1-inch slice of sweet potato, peel, and cut into small pieces. Place in ½-cup glass bowl. Cover with apple juice and microwave, covered, on high for 2½ minutes. Mash, purée, or serve as a finger food.

o o o

Turnips

½ turnip, peeled
1 tbsp. water

Cut turnip into small cubes, and combine with water in 1-cup glass bowl. Cover and cook for 3 minutes on high. Serve as a finger food. For puréeing or mashing, add another 2 minutes cooking time, or until soft.

1 CHILD SERVING

o o o

Zucchini Parmesan

Six ¼-inch slices washed zucchini
½ tsp. butter or margarine
1 tsp. grated Parmesan cheese

Arrange zucchini slices evenly around a microwave-safe plate. Dot with butter or margarine, and sprinkle with Parmesan cheese. Cover with another plate, and microwave on high for 1 minute.

1 CHILD SERVING

o o o

Zucchini and Tomato

½-inch slice zucchini, finely cubed
¼ tomato, cut into small pieces
½ clove garlic, peeled and crushed (optional)

Place zucchini, tomato, and garlic (if desired) in ½-cup glass bowl. Cover and microwave for 1 minute. Cool before serving.

1 CHILD SERVING

o o o

Zucchini, Tomatoes, and Mushrooms

1 tbsp. olive oil
2 cloves garlic, peeled and
    minced
2 cups zucchini, washed and
    cubed
1 ripe tomato, chopped
4 mushrooms, washed and
    sliced

Combine oil and garlic in 4-cup glass bowl, and microwave, uncovered, on high for 1 minute. Add remaining ingredients and mix well. Cover with plate and microwave on high for 2 minutes, stir, and continue cooking for 3 minutes more. Serve with grated Parmesan cheese and chopped parsley.

SERVES 3 TO 4

GRAINS

Corn Bread

1 packet corn bread mix
1 cup milk
2 eggs, beaten
¼ cup vegetable oil

Mix all ingredients, pour into 8 × 8 × 2-inch glass dish. Microwave on medium for 9 minutes, then increase to high for 3 more minutes. Let stand for at least 10 minutes before serving.

APPROXIMATELY 8 SERVINGS

o o o

Couscous (Semolina)

1 tbsp. butter or margarine
¼ cup couscous (found in
   supermarkets and Middle
   Eastern specialty stores)
1 cup water or chicken broth
Mixed Vegetables (see
   below)

Melt butter or margarine in 2-cup bowl and microwave on high for 30 seconds. Stir in couscous. Add water or broth and microwave, uncovered, for 4 to 6 minutes, or until all the liquid is absorbed. Serve with mixed vegetables.

MIXED VEGETABLES

¼ carrot, finely chopped
¼ ripe tomato, finely
   chopped
1½-inch piece of zucchini,
   finely chopped
1 tbsp. raisins
2 tbsp. water

Mix all ingredients in small glass bowl. Cover with plate and microwave on high for 3 minutes. Combine with couscous before serving.

4 CHILD SERVINGS (MAY BE FROZEN)

○ ○ ○

Curried Couscous
(A mildly spiced dish, for toddlers and adults)

2 tbsp. butter or margarine
2 cloves garlic, peeled
¼ small onion
½ tbsp. cumin powder
¼ tsp. curry powder
¼ cup couscous
1 cup chicken broth

Put butter or margarine, garlic, and onion into food processor, and process until finely chopped. Transfer to 8-cup glass bowl and microwave on high for 1 minute. Add cumin and curry powder and continue to cook for another minute. Stir in couscous and chicken broth, and microwave on high, uncovered, for 4 to 6 minutes, or until liquid is absorbed. Serve with mixed vegetables (see recipe on page 317).

SERVES 2

○ ○ ○

Polenta

1 cup water
½ tsp. olive oil
Scant ¼ cup yellow
  cornmeal
¼ cup grated Parmesan
  cheese (optional)

Combine all ingredients, except cheese, in 4-cup glass bowl and cover. Microwave on high for 3 minutes, stirring halfway through. Add cheese, if desired.

SERVES 1

○ ○ ○

Rapid Risotto

1 tbsp. butter or margarine
1 tbsp. olive oil
¼ cup chopped onion
½ cup arborio (Italian) rice

¾ cup chicken broth
  (homemade is best;
  see page 280)
¾ cup water

In 4-cup glass bowl, combine butter or margarine, oil, and onion. Microwave on high for 1 minute. Stir in rice and microwave, uncovered, on high for 2 minutes. Add chicken broth and water and microwave, uncovered, for another 8 minutes on high. Stir, and cook on high for 6 to 8 minutes more, until most of moisture is absorbed. Let stand, uncovered, for 5 minutes. Sprinkle with Parmesan cheese and/or fresh chopped parsley, if desired.

For variation, substitute ¾ cup canned tomatoes with juice,

chopped, in place of chicken broth. Increase water to 1¼ cups. Add 1 clove garlic, peeled and crushed.

SERVES 2

LIGHT MEALS

○ ○ ○

Megan's Favorite Chicken Soup

1 chicken tender, finely
    chopped
2 tbsp. instant or minute rice
    (or very tiny pasta, such
    as orzo)

10 thin carrot slices
1 cup chicken broth
    (preferably homemade
    with no salt; see page 280)

Combine all ingredients in 2-cup bowl, cover with plate, and microwave on high for 5 minutes.

2 CHILD SERVINGS

○ ○ ○

Corn, Crab, and Curry Soup
(An easy, delicious, mild treat)

1 tbsp. butter or margarine
⅓ cup finely chopped onion
14-oz. can chicken broth (or homemade; see page 280)
8 oz. corn (fresh, frozen, or canned)

8 oz. chopped crab (or imitation crab)
1 tsp. mild curry powder (or to taste)
1 cup half-and-half or milk

Place butter or margarine and onion in 8-cup glass bowl. Microwave on high, uncovered, for 3 minutes. Add broth and corn, and cook on high for 5 minutes. Add crab, curry, and half-and-half or milk. Microwave on high for another 3 minutes, or until hot but not boiling.

SERVES 4

○ ○ ○

Simple Cheese Omelet

1 tbsp. butter or margarine
2 eggs, well beaten
2 tbsp. water
½ cup shredded Cheddar cheese

Put butter or margarine into 9-inch glass pie plate and microwave, uncovered, on high for 30 seconds, or until melted. Tilt plate to cover with melted butter. Blend eggs and water together, pour into pie plate, and cook on high for 1 minute.
(continued)

Stir, and cook for 1 minute more. Sprinkle eggs with cheese and cook another 30 seconds on high. Cover and let stand for 1 to 2 minutes until omelet is set and cheese is melted. Fold in half and serve immediately.

SERVES 1

○ ○ ○

Mini "Pizza"

½ English muffin
1½ tbsp. tomato sauce, homemade (see page 283) or canned
2 tbsp. mozzarella cheese, grated

Toast muffin, spread with tomato sauce, and sprinkle with cheese. Microwave on high for 1 minute, until cheese is melted.

1 CHILD SERVING

○ ○ ○

Tortilla to Go

¼ cup Cheddar cheese, grated
1 small tortilla (corn or flour)

Sprinkle cheese on tortilla, and place tortilla on microwave-safe plate. Cook on high, uncovered, for 30 to 40 seconds, or until cheese is melted. (Do not overcook.)

SERVES 1

○ ○ ○

Creamed Chicken on Toast

1 tbsp. butter or margarine
1 tbsp. flour
1 cup milk
5-oz. can white-meat
   chicken, drained, rinsed,
   and chopped, or 3 cooked
   chicken tenders, chopped
4 slices whole wheat toast

Melt butter or margarine in 4-cup glass bowl. Mix in flour and milk with a wire whisk. Microwave, uncovered, for 4 minutes on high, stirring once, until sauce has thickened. Arrange chicken on toast slices, and cover with white sauce.

SERVES 4

○ ○ ○

Chicken Rice Cake Crunch

1 chicken tender, cooked or
   2 oz. canned chicken, well
   rinsed
1 tbsp. light mayonnaise
¼ tsp. dill

Pinch celery seed
4 cucumber slices, peeled
1 rice cake

Combine chicken, mayonnaise, and spices. Arrange cucumber slices on rice cake, and top with chicken mixture.

SERVES 1

o o o

Stuffed Potato au Gratin

1 medium baked potato (see page 311)
¼ cup Cheddar cheese
¼ cup cooked broccoli florets (optional)

Split cooked potato lengthwise, sprinkle with cheese (over broccoli, if used), and microwave on high for 45 seconds, or until cheese is melted.

SERVES 1

MAIN MEALS

Mild Curried Fish

½ medium onion, peeled and thinly sliced
1 cup celery, washed and finely chopped
1 tsp. curry powder
1 tbsp. butter or margarine

¼ cup milk
1 lb. orange roughy, fresh or defrosted
1 tbsp. lemon juice

In 2-cup bowl, combine onion, celery, curry powder, and butter or margarine. Cover and microwave on high for 3 minutes. Add milk and stir until well mixed. Place fish in 8 × 8 × 2-inch glass dish, sprinkle with lemon juice, add vegetable mixture, cover, and microwave on high for 7 minutes. Let stand 3 minutes before serving.

SERVES 3

○ ○ ○

Fillet of Sole Tarragon

¼ cup onion   1 tsp. dry tarragon
1 tbsp. butter or margarine   ¼ cup dry white wine
1 lb. sole fillets, fresh or
   defrosted
1 tbsp. lemon juice

Combine onion and butter or margarine in small glass bowl
and microwave on high for 3 minutes. Meanwhile, place sole
in 8×8×2-inch glass dish. Sprinkle with lemon juice and tarragon. Cover with onion mixture and white wine. Cover and
microwave on high for 6 minutes. Let stand 5 minutes before
serving.

SERVES 3

○ ○ ○

Basic Poached Chicken Breast

1 boneless, skinless chicken breast
2 tbsp. lemon juice, white wine, chicken broth, or sherry

Place chicken breast between 2 sheets of wax paper and flatten
with mallet. Remove from paper and place on flat microwave-safe
dish. Pour liquid over chicken. Cover and microwave for 2 minutes on high. Turn and microwave for an additional 2 minutes.

SERVES 1

SAUCES TO SERVE WITH POACHED CHICKEN

MUSHROOM CREAM SAUCE

1 tbsp. butter or margarine
1 tbsp. chopped onion
1 tbsp. chopped mushrooms
1 clove garlic, crushed
1 tbsp. flour

½ cup chicken broth
   (homemade preferably;
   see page 280)
¼ cup half-and-half or milk
1 tbsp. lemon juice
2 tbsp. sherry (optional)

In 2-cup glass bowl microwave butter or margarine, onion, mushrooms, and garlic for 1 minute on high, uncovered. Remove from oven, stir in flour until well blended. Slowly whisk in chicken broth, half-and-half, lemon juice, and sherry, if desired. Microwave on high, uncovered, for 3 minutes, stirring halfway through. If liquid seems too thick, add a little extra broth for the right consistency.

For variation, add ¼ cup of cooked broccoli to sauce, spoon over chicken breast, and heat for 30 to 40 seconds on high before serving.

MUSHROOM SAUCE WITH MUSTARD AND GINGER

Following Mushroom Cream Sauce recipe, add ½ tsp. Dijon mustard and ½ tsp. ground ginger to sauce, and cook on high for 30 seconds.

LEEK AND TOMATO SAUCE

1 tbsp. butter or margarine
½ tsp. peeled and crushed
  garlic
1 tbsp. lemon juice
¼ cup leek, well washed
  and thinly sliced

2 tbsp. chopped tomatoes
2 tbsp. sherry (optional)
¼ cup chicken broth
   (homemade preferably;
   see page 280)

In 2-cup glass bowl, combine butter or margarine, garlic, lemon juice, and leek. Microwave, uncovered, on high for 2 minutes. Add tomatoes, sherry, if desired, and chicken broth, and continue to microwave for 2 more minutes on high. Stir, and pour over chicken breast. Heat both in microwave for 30 to 40 seconds on high, if needed.

VEGETABLE WINE SAUCE

2 tbsp. butter or margarine
2 tbsp. onion, peeled and
  finely chopped
1 clove garlic, peeled and
  crushed
2 tbsp. mushrooms, sliced
  or chopped
2 tbsp. celery, chopped

2 tbsp. red pepper, chopped
2 tbsp. thinly sliced leek
¼ cup chicken broth
  (homemade preferably;
  see page 280)
¼ cup white wine

In 2-cup glass bowl, combine butter, or margarine, onion, and garlic, and microwave, uncovered, on high for 2 minutes. Add mushrooms, celery, red pepper, and leek, and cook on high for 2 minutes more. Add broth and wine, and microwave, uncovered, for 5 minutes on high. Pour over chicken, and heat for another 30 seconds, if needed.

LIGHT TOMATO SAUCE

1 tbsp. butter or margarine
1 tbsp. onion, peeled and
  finely chopped
1 clove garlic, peeled and
  crushed
2 tbsp. tomato sauce, or 1
  tsp. tomato paste

1 tbsp. sherry
¼ cup half-and-half or milk

In 2-cup glass bowl, combine butter or margarine, onion, and garlic. Microwave, uncovered, for 1 minute on high. Add tomato sauce, sherry, and half-and-half or milk. Microwave, uncovered, on high for 1 more minute. Pour over chicken and heat for 30 seconds, if needed. Garnish with parsley, if desired.

These sauces also work well over fish, meat patties, or even pasta.

o o o

Chicken Fricassee

1 tbsp. butter or margarine
1 tbsp. flour
1 cup chicken broth (homemade preferably; see page 280)
2 chicken tenders, finely diced
¼ carrot, scrubbed and finely diced

¼ potato, peeled and finely diced
1 caulifloweret, broken into small pieces
1 tbsp. frozen tiny peas
¼ cup chicken broth or water

Melt butter or margarine in 2-cup glass bowl for 30 seconds. Mix in flour with wire whisk, add 1 cup of chicken broth, stir, and microwave on high for 5 minutes, stirring once. While sauce is cooking, put chicken and all vegetables into a 1-cup glass bowl, add ¼ cup of chicken broth or water, cover with plate, and microwave on high for 3 minutes. Add these ingredients to the sauce, mix well, cover, and microwave on high for 1 more minute. Stir again, and serve.

2 CHILD SERVINGS

o o o

Chicken and Brown Rice

½ cup water
1 tsp. butter or margarine
¼ cup instant brown rice
1 chicken tender, cut into
    tiny pieces
1 tbsp. red bell pepper,
    finely chopped
1 tbsp. green bell pepper,
    finely chopped

Place water, butter or margarine, and rice in 2-cup glass bowl, and microwave on high for 5 minutes. Add all remaining ingredients, cover, and cook on high for 1 more minute. Let stand for 2 to 5 minutes, or until liquid is absorbed.

1 TODDLER SERVING

o o o

Turkey Ragout

½ lb. ground turkey
2 medium potatoes, peeled
    and thinly sliced
¼ tsp. garlic powder
½ tsp. paprika

1 tbsp. parsley flakes
2 medium carrots, scrubbed
    and sliced
4 tbsp. water

Form turkey into six small, round, flat patties. Place in 8×8×2-inch glass dish and cover with sliced potatoes. Sprinkle half the garlic powder, paprika, and parsley flakes over potatoes, add a layer of carrots, and sprinkle remaining garlic,

paprika, and parsley. Add water to dish, cover, and microwave on medium high for 12 minutes. Let stand for 5 minutes
before serving.

SERVES 3

o o o

In Defense of Meatloaf

½ cup bread crumbs
1 cup low-fat or nonfat milk
1 lb. ground turkey or extra-
  lean ground beef
1 small onion, minced
2 eggs, beaten

2 tsp. sage (optional)
1 tbsp. dried parsley flakes
⅓ cup tomato sauce or
  ketchup
Piquante Sauce to cover
  (recipe follows)

Soak bread crumbs in milk. Mix all other ingredients (except
piquante sauce) well and add milk and bread crumb mixture.
Form loaf in glass or ceramic bread pan. Spread half of piquante sauce evenly over top, cover, and microwave on medium high for 21 to 23 minutes. Remove and let stand 5
minutes. Cover with remaining piquante sauce and microwave on high for 5 minutes more. (For cooking in conventional oven, bake at 350°F for 1 hour.)

SERVES 4

o o o

Piquante Sauce

½ cup ketchup
2 tsp. dry mustard
5 tsp. brown sugar

Mix well.

SERVES 4

o o o

Quick Chili

8 oz. ground turkey or lean
  ground beef
½ cup chopped onion
¼ tsp. garlic powder
¼ tsp. chili powder, or to
  taste

1 tsp. ground cumin
16-oz. can tomatoes,
  chopped
1 cup kidney beans, canned
  or precooked
8-oz. can tomato sauce

Crumble ground turkey or beef into a 4-cup glass bowl, add onion and garlic powder, and microwave on high for 3 minutes. Stir well, add chili powder and cumin, tomatoes, kidney beans, and tomato sauce. Mix again, cover with plate, and microwave on high for another 12 minutes. Serve with shredded cheese, sliced ripe olives (if desired), and corn bread (see page 248) or oyster crackers.

MAKES 4 ONE-CUP SERVINGS

o o o

Cottage Pie

1 lb. extra-lean ground beef
  or ground turkey
½ tsp. paprika
½ tsp. garlic powder
¼ tsp. pepper

4 cups mashed potatoes
1 cup grated cheese
  (Cheddar, jack, or
  mozzarella)

Put meat into 8-cup glass pan, sprinkle with the spices, cover, and cook on high for 6 minutes, stirring halfway through. Remove meat and cover with layer of mashed potatoes, then add grated cheese. Cover. Microwave on high for 10 minutes, or until cheese is melted. Serve with broccoli, peas, or green beans.

    This is an excellent way to use up leftover mashed potatoes. Alternatively, boil 4 large potatoes conventionally and mash well, or use instant potatoes (which are not so tasty, but are very quick to prepare).

SERVES 3 TO 4

o o o

Basic Alphabet Pasta with Vegetables

1 cup water
1 tbsp. alphabet, pastina, or
  stelline (stars) pasta*
1 tbsp. chopped fresh
  zucchini

1 tbsp. chopped fresh
  tomato
½ tbsp. Parmesan cheese
  (optional)

*Larger pastas take too long to cook in the microwave.

Microwave water in 2-cup bowl for 2½ to 3 minutes on high, uncovered, until water boils. Immediately add pasta, stir, and microwave for another 10 minutes on high. (Approximately 1 tablespoonful of liquid should remain. If there is more, cook pasta for another minute or two.) Remove from oven, stir in vegetables, cover with a plate, and microwave on high for 1 minute. Let stand for 5 minutes. Sprinkle with Parmesan cheese, if desired, and serve.

This dish adapts beautifully to a variety of pleasing meals. Following the basics above, try one of these variations:

- Substitute green beans, peas, carrots, or other simple vegetables, cut into small pieces, for zucchini and tomato. Increase cooking time to 2 minutes, if necessary.
- Top pasta with a tablespoonful of homemade tomato sauce (see page 283), or canned.
- Finely dice a chicken tender and cook with pasta for 1 minute. Mix with vegetables and/or 2 tbsp. tomato sauce.
- Microwave 1 tbsp. extra-lean ground beef or ground turkey for 1 minute. Mix with 3 tbsp. tomato sauce and pour over pasta.
- Toss pasta with ½ tsp. butter or margarine, and sprinkle with 1 tbsp. grated cheese (almost any mild cheese).
- Blend 1 tbsp. cottage or ricotta cheese with pasta and vegetables.
- Mix with 2 tbsp. finely chopped cooked spinach.

1 CHILD SERVING

DESSERTS

o o o

Apple or Pear

½ sweet apple or ripe pear, peeled and cored

Cut fruit into thirds, place on microwave-safe dish, and cook on high for 30 seconds. May be puréed or mashed.

1 CHILD SERVING

o o o

Microwave Baked Apples

4 small or medium apples
   (Rome or Delicious are
   best), washed
4 tsp. butter or margarine

4 tsp. brown sugar
   (optional)
¼ cup water

Core apples, removing all seeds, but do not pierce bottoms. Fill each apple with 1 tsp. butter or margarine and brown sugar, if desired. Place apples evenly around a glass pie dish, add water, and cover with wax paper. Microwave on high for 5 minutes, or until apple is soft.

SERVES 4

o o o

Banana with Chocolate Sauce

2 bananas, peeled and
   halved
1 tbsp. butter or margarine,
   melted
1 oz. (1 square) semisweet
   chocolate
1 tsp. vegetable shortening

Place banana halves in glass pie plate, dribble melted butter
or margarine over each piece, and microwave on high for 1
minute. In a small glass bowl, combine chocolate and vegetable shortening, and microwave on high for 1 minute. Stir well.
If not completely melted, microwave for another 30 seconds,
or until chocolate is melted. Put half a banana on each dish
and drizzle a little chocolate sauce over.

SERVES 4

o o o

Cooked Fruit

½ large plum (3 inches), nectarine, or peach

Rinse fruit, slice, pit, and place cut-side down on microwave-
safe plate. Microwave on high for 1 minute. Remove peel,
mash or purée, and cool before serving.

1 CHILD SERVING

o o o

Fruit Compote

1 pear, cored and cubed
1 orange, peeled and cut
    into bite-size pieces
¼ cup fresh or dried
    apricots, rinsed and
    chopped
¼ cup pitted prunes
⅓ cup orange juice

Place all ingredients in 4-cup glass bowl. Cover with plate and microwave on high for 5 minutes. Serve with half-and-half, if desired.

SERVES 3

o o o

Pastry Shells
(Can be made in conventional oven)

½ cup all-purpose flour
2 tbsp. vegetable shortening
⅛ tsp. salt
1 tbsp. plus 2 tsp. cold water

In small bowl combine flour, shortening, and salt. Using a fork, blend until mixture is crumbly. Mix in 1 tbsp. of water with fork, then use hands to blend completely. Dough should hold together. If necessary, add up to 2 tsp. more water. Roll out dough to less than ⅛-inch thick and, using small glass bowl or custard cup, press into pastry to make rounds. Insert pastry into bowl or cup, press down lightly, prick bottom of shell several times with fork, and microwave on high for 1½ minutes.

For conventional oven, use a metal-cup cake pan and bake at 375°F for 15 minutes.

May be filled with fresh or cooked berries and other fruit, or with creamed chicken or vegetables for a main course or side dish.

MAKES 1 LARGE OR 2 SMALL SHELLS

○ ○ ○

Creamy Rice Pudding

2 cups cooked white or
   brown rice
½ cup raisins
2 cups milk
1 tbsp. vegetable oil
1 tsp. vanilla extract

Combine rice and raisins in 4-cup glass bowl. Whisk together remaining ingredients and mix with rice. Cover, and microwave on medium for 30 minutes. Stir before serving.

SERVES 3 TO 4

o o o

Veiled Maidens

⅓ cup butter or margarine
1½ cups graham cracker
   crumbs
2 tbsp. sugar
Raspberry Sauce (see below)

Place butter or margarine in 9-inch glass pie plate. Microwave on high for 1 or 2 minutes, until melted. Stir in graham cracker crumbs and sugar. Press crumb mixture into pie plate to make a crust. Microwave on high for 1½ to 2 minutes more, or until set. Cool, and fill with raspberry sauce.

RASPBERRY SAUCE

1 cup fresh raspberries
1 tbsp. sugar
½ tsp. lemon juice

Combine raspberries, sugar, and lemon juice in food processor, and blend for 10 seconds or until well mixed. Pour sauce into pie crust. Top with whipped cream, if desired.

For variation make an applesauce. Core, peel, and chop 4 sweet apples. Microwave in 4-cup glass bowl on high for 3 to 4 minutes, or until soft. Purée with sugar and lemon juice in food processor, and proceed as for raspberry sauce.

SERVES 4 TO 6

SAUCES

o o o

Easy "Scratch" Chicken Broth

4 cups water
2 pieces chicken breast or
  thighs
1 stalk celery, washed and
  cut into thirds
2 small onions, peeled and
  quartered
1 or 2 carrots, washed and
  halved

1 clove garlic, peeled and
  crushed
1 bay leaf
1 small handful fresh
  parsley
1 tbsp. whole peppercorn
1 tsp. salt (optional)

Place all ingredients in 8-cup glass bowl. Cover with plate and
microwave on medium high for 30 minutes. Remove from
oven carefully, strain liquid through sieve, and cool. Defat if
necessary.

Note: Many soup and sauce recipes call for chicken broth.
Homemade is recommended, as canned broth usually contains a lot of salt and MSG.

○ ○ ○

Microwave Tomato Sauce

2 garlic cloves, peeled and
  crushed
1 small onion, peeled and
  finely chopped
2 tbsp. olive oil
28-oz. can crushed
  tomatoes, with added
  purée

3 oz. tomato paste
14 oz. water
1 tbsp. oregano
1 tbsp. basil

In 8-cup glass bowl, mix garlic and onion with olive oil, cover bowl with plate, and microwave on high for 5 minutes. Add all other ingredients, stir, cover, and microwave for 30 minutes on medium high.

This sauce freezes well, and can be stored in small portions for many dishes.

○ ○ ○

Speedy Hot Bean Dip

16-oz. can refried beans
3-oz. can mild Ortega green
  chilies, diced
¾ cup Cheddar cheese,
  shredded
½ cup jack cheese, shredded

Mix all ingredients well, place in 4-cup glass dish, and cover. Microwave on medium for 8 minutes, or until cheese is melted.

This makes a good spread for toddlers, on rice cakes, tortillas, or crackers. For older children and adults, use as a dip with corn chips, carrot sticks, or as an accompaniment to Mexican-style dishes.

Crockpot Cooking

In tandem with the microwave oven, the crockpot is a wonderful time-saver for busy parents. Although a large variety of dishes cook well and quickly in the microwave, many meals benefit from long, slow cooking and cannot be microwaved successfully.

By quickly preparing the ingredients the day before, you can literally toss them into the crockpot before leaving in the morning and come home to a delicious, ready-to-serve meal that has been cooking slowly all day. Besides the obvious benefits, crockpot cooking enables all the nutrients in foods to be retained. In addition, meats become very tender, and are ideal for puréeing or cutting up for young children. And the aroma you come home to is wonderful!

FAMILY RECIPES

Crockpot Seafood Chowder

1 lb. frozen cod, slightly thawed and cut into bite-size pieces
2 potatoes, peeled and diced
1 small onion, peeled and chopped
1 small bell pepper, chopped
½ cup celery, chopped
½ cup carrots, sliced
¼ cup fresh parsley, chopped

16-oz. can tomatoes, cut up
1½ cups water
1 tbsp. olive oil
1 tsp. dried basil
½ tsp. dried thyme
⅛ tsp. ground black pepper
⅓ cup sherry (optional)
⅛ tsp. dried red chili pepper (optional)

Combine all ingredients in crockpot and cover. Cook on low for 9 hours, or on high for 3½ hours, until potatoes are tender.

SERVES 4 TO 6

o o o

Crockpot Chicken Soup

2 chicken breast halves, or 4
    thighs, skinned
4 carrots, scrubbed and cut
    into 1-inch slices
4 potatoes, scrubbed or
    peeled and quartered, or
    ¼ cup rice
1 medium onion, peeled and
    chopped
2 celery stalks, cut into 1-
    inch pieces

1 clove garlic, peeled and
    crushed
¼ cup fresh parsley,
    chopped, or 3 tbsp. dried
    parsley
14½ oz. chicken broth,
    canned or homemade (see
    page 280)
1 cup water

Place all ingredients in crockpot and cook on low for 8 to 10
hours, or on high for 3½ to 5 hours.

Noodles may be substituted for potatoes or rice. Add 1 cup
cooked noodles in last half hour of cooking. Alternatively, add
1 cup uncooked noodles to crockpot for last hour, and turn
temperature to high.

SERVES 4

o o o

Crockpot Split Pea Soup

2 cups split peas (soaked
    overnight, drained, and
    rinsed)
1 medium onion, peeled and
    chopped
1 cup celery, chopped
1 cup carrots, chopped

1 bay leaf
½ tsp. thyme
Water to cover

(continued)

Combine all ingredients in crockpot and stir. Cover and cook on low for 10 to 12 hours, or on high for 5 to 6 hours.

SERVES 6 TO 8

o o o

Crockpot Chicken with Tarragon and Wine*

1½ tbsp. dried tarragon
½ tsp. pepper
1 whole frying or roasting
   chicken, well rinsed
½ cup dry white wine
½ cup chicken broth
   (homemade preferably;
   see page 280)

Rub tarragon and pepper on outside and inside of chicken. Place in crockpot, cover with liquids, and cook on low for 8 to 10 hours, or on high for 4 to 6 hours.

SERVES 4

*Alcohol in wine completely evaporates during cooking.

o o o

Crockpot Chicken and Dumplings

2 whole skinned chicken breasts, or 4 skinned thighs
4 carrots, scrubbed and cut into 1-inch pieces
2 celery stalks, cut into 1-inch pieces
½ medium onion, peeled
14½-oz. can chicken broth, or homemade (see page 280)

2 cups water
¼ cup chopped fresh parsley or 3 tbsp. dried parsley
1 clove garlic, peeled and crushed
¼ tsp. pepper
½ tsp. salt (optional)

Combine all ingredients in crockpot, mix well, cover, and cook on low for 8 to 10 hours, or on high for 4 to 6 hours.

Dumplings

1 cup flour
⅓ cup green onion, finely chopped
2 tbsp. finely chopped fresh parsley, or 1 tbsp. dried parsley

1¼ tsp. baking powder
¼ tsp. salt
2 tbsp. butter or margarine, chilled
½ cup milk

Mix all ingredients, except butter or margarine and milk, in a bowl. Cut in butter or margarine until mixture has a uniform crumblike texture. Stir in milk until evenly moistened. Cover with cloth and refrigerate until ready to cook.

Forty-five minutes before chicken is finished in crockpot, remove onion from pot. Using a tablespoon, make small dumplings from dough, and drop on top of chicken in crockpot. Cook for 45 minutes to 1 hour on high. (The dumplings should be large and fluffy.)

Microwave Dumplings

Using the recipe on page 345 remove 1 cup of liquid from crockpot and add to 4-cup bowl with dumplings. Cover and microwave on high for 8 minutes. Return dumplings to crock-pot chicken and serve.

SERVES 4

o o o

Crockpot Chicken, Beans, and Sausage

4 chicken thighs, or 3
  chicken breast halves,
  skinned
8 oz. turkey or breakfast
  sausage, cut into 2-inch
  pieces
1 medium onion, peeled and
  quartered

4 medium carrots, scrubbed
  and halved
16-oz. can white beans
1 cup white wine*
½ tsp. thyme
1 bay leaf

Place all ingredients in crockpot, mix, and cover. Cook on low for 8 to 10 hours, or on high for 4 hours.

SERVES 4

*Alcohol will completely evaporate during cooking.

○ ○ ○

Crockpot Baked Potatoes

6 baking potatoes

Scrub potatoes well, and prick in 2 or 3 places with a fork. Seal in foil, and place in crockpot. Cook on low for 8 to 10 hours, or on high for 2½ to 4 hours. (Do not add water.)

SERVES 6

○ ○ ○

Crockpot BBQ Ribs and Baked Potatoes

4 baking potatoes, scrubbed
3 lbs. spareribs
1 cup barbecue sauce (homemade or store-bought)

Prick potatoes twice with fork, seal in foil, and place in bottom of crockpot. Place ribs over potatoes, cover with barbecue sauce, and cook for 8 to 10 hours on low, or for 4 to 5 hours on high.

SERVES 4

○ ○ ○

Crockpot Curry

2 lbs. boneless lamb, cut
   into 1-inch cubes (chicken
   may be substituted)
1 large onion, peeled and
   chopped
2 stalks celery, chopped
½ cup raisins
3 oz. tomato paste
1½ cups stock or water

2 tbsp. curry powder
¼ tsp. pepper
¼ tsp. turmeric
½ tsp. cumin
½ tsp. coriander
1 bay leaf

Combine all ingredients in crockpot, mix well, and cover.
Cook on low for 8 to 9 hours, or on high for 4 to 5 hours.
Serve with rice.

SERVES 4 TO 6

○ ○ ○

Crockpot Boeuf à la Mode

1 large onion, peeled and
   sliced
1 cup celery, sliced
2 cups carrots, scrubbed and
   sliced
2-lb. rump pot roast, all fat
   removed
2 cloves garlic (unpeeled),
   halved
¼ cup minced parsley, or 2
   tbsp. dried parsley

¼ tsp. pepper
1 bay leaf
¾ cup chicken or vegetable
   stock (see page 280 or
   page 281)
1 cup red wine (chicken or
   beef broth may be
   substituted)
¼ cup water and olive oil,
   combined

Place onion, celery, and half the carrots on bottom of crockpot. Add roast, spices, and all liquid. Cover with remaining carrots, and cook on low for 10 to 12 hours, or on high for 5 to 6 hours. Serve with wide noodles.

SERVES 4 TO 6

o o o

Crockpot Corned Beef and Cabbage

3-lb. corned beef brisket
  (packed with spices)
4 potatoes, peeled and
  halved
3 carrots, scrubbed and cut
  into thirds

2 small onions, peeled and
  quartered
1 cup water
½ head cabbage, washed
  and quartered

Combine all ingredients, except cabbage, in crockpot, cover, and cook on low for 8 to 10 hours, or on high for 5 to 6 hours. Add cabbage during last 2 hours on low, or last 1 hour on high, if possible. Otherwise, cabbage may be microwaved as follows: Arrange quarters evenly around a shallow microwaveable dish, with core edges toward the middle. Cover and microwave for 12 minutes on high. Add to crockpot.

Note: It is good to make this meal a day ahead, cool, and defat.

SERVES 4

o˙o o

Crockpot Beef Stew

¼ cup flour
1 lb. lean beef, cut into 1-
    inch cubes
4 carrots, scrubbed and cut
    into ½-inch slices
4 potatoes, peeled and
    cubed
1 small onion, peeled and
    finely chopped

1 celery stalk, cut into
    ½-inch slices
1 clove garlic, peeled and
    crushed
1 bay leaf
1½ cups water or chicken
    broth (homemade
    preferably; see page 280)

Stir flour with meat to cover. Place in crockpot. Add all remaining ingredients, mix well, and cook on low for 10 to 12
hours, or on high for 4 to 6 hours.

SERVES 4

References

Composition of Foods—Raw, Processed, Prepared (Agricultural Handbook No. 8), by Bernice K. Watt and Annabel L. Merrill. Washington, D.C.: U.S. Department of Agriculture, Agricultural Research Service, 1963.

Diet Manual Massachusetts General Hospital. Boston: Little, Brown, 1976.

Essentials of Nutrition and Diet Therapy by Sue Rodwell Williams. St. Louis: The C. V. Mosby Company, 1974.

Maternal and Child Nutrition: Assessment and Counseling by Jill S. Slattery, et al., eds. New York: Appleton-Century-Crofts, 1979.

Nutrition in Infancy and Childhood by Peggy L. Pipes. St. Louis: The C. V. Mosby Company, 1977.

Pediatric Nutrition Handbook. Evanston, Ill.: American Academy of Pediatrics, 1979.

Recommended Dietary Allowances. Washington, D.C.: Food and Nutrition Board, National Academy of Sciences, National Research Council, Revised 1989.

We are indebted to the following authors from whose books we have adapted recipes and cooking methods for the special purposes of *The Baby Cookbook, Revised Edition.*

Atwater, Maxine. *Natural Foods Cookbook.* Concord, Calif.: Nitty Gritty Productions, 1972.

Cottrell, Edith Young. *The Oats, Peas, Beans and Barley Cookbook.* Santa Barbara, Calif.: Woodbridge Press, 1974.

Hunter, Beatrice Trum. *The Natural Foods Cookbook.* New York: Simon & Schuster, 1961.

Wilson, Ellen Gibson. *A West African Cook Book.* New York: M. Evans, 1971.

Zane, Eva. *Middle Eastern Cookery.* San Francisco: 101 Productions, 1974.

General Index

allergies, food, 61–62, 63, 64, 98
American Academy of Pediatrics, 28, 31,
  50, 57, 63
American Academy of Pedodontists,
  57
amino acids, 22–23, 73
anemia, 62, 104
appetite, 49, 60, 75, 108, 126, 127
  overeating and, 102–103
  poor, reasons for, 107, 108, 121
  tooth decay and, 56
  weather and, 127
apple juice, 99
apples, 65
apricots, 65
arteriosclerosis, 27
ascorbic acid, see vitamin C
avocado, 105–106

baby foods, commercial:
  iron lacking in, 46
  reading labels on, 73, 98
baby foods, homemade, 68–71
  advantages of, 68
  cereals, 69–70
  equipment needed for, 69, 71
  fish, 70
  freezing of, 76
  fruits, 70, 71
  meats, 70, 71
  points to remember when preparing,
    68–69
  saving time in, 71
  vegetables, 70, 71
bananas, 65, 98, 109
barley, 96, 97

beans, 29, 109
  lima, 109
  protein in, 23
  see also legumes
beef, 65
beta carotene, 35, 45
BHA and BHT, 73
biotin, 35, 36
blacks, lactose intolerance in, 51
blackstrap molasses, 55
bottle feeding, 64, 104
  feeding solids before vs. after, 63
  as pacifier, 56
  to quiet baby, 60
  tooth decay and, 56–57, 65, 96
  see also formulas, baby
bottle-mouth syndrome, 56–57, 104
botulism, 55, 124
bowel movements:
  diarrhea and, 102, 120
  fruit and, 65
boys, percentile standards for growth in,
  110
brain growth, 112
bran, 131
breads, 29, 61, 93
  fiber in, 31, 32–33
  making of, 130–131
  white vs. whole-grain, 131
breakfast menus, 72–75, 99
breast feeding, see nursing
breast milk, see milk, breast
brewer's yeast, 73, 108
broccoli, 106, 109
brown sugar, 55
butter, 27, 50, 54

RECIPE INDEX

*Special recipes for babies and
toddlers in this index
are in* **boldface type.**